KEY QUESTION

OBSTETRICS AND GYNAECOLOGY

Second Edition

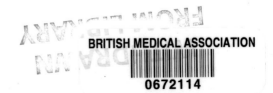

Also of interest:

Key Topics in Obstetrics and Gynaecology, 2nd edition
R. Slade, E. Laird, G. Beynon and A. Pickersgill
Publication date January 1998

ISBN 1 85996 226 2

KEY QUESTIONS IN
OBSTETRICS AND GYNAECOLOGY

Second Edition

A. PICKERSGILL
MRCOG
Lecturer in Obstetrics and Gynaecology, University of Manchester, Manchester, UK

A. MESKHI
MRCOG
Senior SHO in Obstetrics and Gynaecology, Huddersfield Royal Infirmary, Huddersfield, UK

S. PAUL
MRCOG, MD
Specialist Registrar in Obstetrics and Gynaecology, Arrowe Park Hospital, Wirral, UK

βIOS
SCIENTIFIC
PUBLISHERS

Oxford • Washington DC

© BIOS Scientific Publishers Limited, 1999

First published 1994
Second edition published 1999
Reprinted 2002

A CIP catalogue record for this book is available from the British Library.

ISBN 1 85996 003 0

BIOS Scientific Publishers Ltd
9 Newtec Place, Magdalen Road, Oxford OX4 1RE, UK
Tel. +44 (0)1865 726286. Fax. +44 (0)1865 246823
World Wide Web home page: http://www.bios.co.uk/

Important Note from the Publisher
The information contained within this book was obtained by BIOS Scientific
Publishers Ltd from sources believed by us to be reliable. However, while every effort
has been made to ensure its accuracy, no responsibility for loss or injury whatsoever
occasioned to any person acting or refraining from action as a result of information
contained herein can be accepted by the author's or publishers.

The reader should remember that medicine is a constantly evolving science and while
the authors and publishers have ensured that all dosages, applications and practices
are based on current indications, there may be specific practices which differ between
communities. You should always follow the guidelines laid down by the
manufacturers of specific products and the relevant authorities in the country in which
you are practising.

Production Editor: Fran Kingston
Typeset by Marksbury Multimedia Ltd., Midsomer Norton, Bath, UK
Printed and bound in Great Britain by Biddles Ltd, *www.biddles.co.uk*

CONTENTS

ABBREVIATIONS

AFP	alpha-fetoprotein
APTT	activated partial thromboplastin time
ARDS	adult respiratory distress syndrome
CIN	cervical intraepithelial neoplasia
CPD	cephalo-pelvic disproportion
CT	computerized tomography
CVS	chorionic villus sampling
D&C	dilatation and curettage
DVT	deep vein thrombosis
ELA	endometrial laser ablation
ECV	external cephalic version
FDP	fibrin degradation products
FSH	follicle-stimulating hormone
FTA	fluorescent treponemal antibody
GnRH	gonadotrophin-releasing hormone
G-6-PD	glucose-6-phosphate dehydrogenase
GSI	genuine stress incontinence
GTN	glyceryl trinitrate
GTT	glucose tolerance test
HCG	human chorionic gonadotrophin
HDL	high density lipoprotein
HFEA	Human Fertilisation and Embryology Authority
HIV	human immunodeficiency virus
HPV	human papilloma virus
HRT	hormone replacement therapy
INR	international normalized ratio
IUCD	intrauterine contraceptive device
IUD	intrauterine death
IUGR	intrauterine growth restriction
IV	intravenous
IVP	intravenous pyelogram
LDL	low density lipoprotein
LH	luteinizing hormone
LLETZ	large loop excision of the transformation zone
LNG-IUD	levonorgestrel-releasing intrauterine device
LUF	luteinized unruptured follicle
MCH	mean cell haemoglobin
MCHC	mean cell haemoglobin concentration
MCV	mean cell volume
MRI	magnetic resonance imaging
mRNA	messenger RNA
MSAFP	maternal serum alpha-fetoprotein
MSSU	midstream specimen of urine

OHSS	ovarian hyperstimulation syndrome
PCOS	polycystic ovarian syndrome
PID	pelvic inflammatory disease
PIH	pregnancy-induced hypertension
PMR	perinatal mortality rate
POP	progesterone only pill
PT	prothrombin time
RDS	respiratory distress syndrome
RIF	right iliac fossa
SCBU	special care baby unit
SHBG	sex hormone-binding globulin
SL	sublingual
SLE	systemic lupus erythematosus
T4	thyroxine
T3	triiodothyronine
TCRE	transcervical resection of endometrium
TORCH	toxoplasma, rubella, cytomegalovirus, herpes
UTI	urinary tract infection
VDRL	venereal disease reference laboratory
VIN	vulvar intraepithelial neoplasia

FOREWORD

It gives me great pleasure to write a foreword to the second edition of *Key Questions in Obstetrics and Gynaecology*. It is always much more difficult to write and develop multiple choice questions than it is to do a factual text. The authors should be congratulated on making such an excellent addition to the series and I am sure it will help and encourage many obstetricians and gynaecologists in training to further their careers.

RJ Slade FRCS, MRCOG
Consultant Gynaecological Surgeon

PREFACE

THE EXAMINATION

Despite the recent changes in the Part 2 MRCOG, multiple choice questions (MCQ) remain as an integral component of the written examination and there are no plans to remove them at present.

The examination is divided into an initial written paper (MCQ and short essays) and for those successful, an OSCE. Fixed pass marks apply for both parts of the examination. A mark of 175/300 must be achieved in the written paper, made up of 100/200 in the essay papers and 75/100 in the MCQ (as there is no negative marking this is equivalent to 50%). It is not necessary to achieve 50% in both the essays and the MCQ, merely an overall mark. Candidates proceeding to the oral component of the examination must then achieve a pass mark of 60% to pass the whole of the examination. The MCQ paper consists of 300 questions, to be completed within 2 hours. The questions are in a Question Book and are in the form of a statement (stem) followed by the questions. There may be only one statement and question. For example:

1.   Induction of labour is the artificial initiation of cervical dilation and effacement leading to progressive uterine contractions.

Or one statement followed by multiple answers. For example:

With regard to induction of labour

2.   Vaginal prostaglandins are recommended initially for all women
3. PGF_2 is the prostaglandin of choice and should be used at 6-hourly intervals
4.   Syntocinon should be started at the time of amniotomy
5.   The total dosage should not exceed 4 mg in a multiparous patient
6.   With prelabour rupture of the membranes, prostaglandins improve the outcome
7.   Should not be performed before 41 weeks gestation

An Answer Sheet (see over) is provided separately. On the Answer Sheet each question (1–300) is represented by it's respective number and is followed by 'True' or 'False'. When you have decided on your answer you need to boldly black out the 'lozenge' that represents your answer with the pencil provided. The Answer Sheet is optically read by a document-reading machine (scanner) so care is needed when completing it.

Some candidates prefer to mark True or False in the Question Book as they answer the questions. Care must then be taken when transferring the answers across to the Answer Sheet as mistakes can be made in transcription. We would advise lightly blocking in your answers on the answer sheet as you go along, and then boldly marking over them at the end. Lightly marking the answers allows them to be easily erased (so no smudges can spoil your score) and prevents transcription errors.

The examination is no longer negatively marked. For each correct answer you will score one mark and for each wrong answer (or no response) no marks. Therefore, it is important to answer all of the questions even if you are unsure of the answer. It has been found that the first answer a participant chooses to an MCQ is often the correct one, so if uncertain do not alter your answers.

THE BOOK

The questions in this second edition of the book are completely new and have been written in a similar format to the new style of examination questions. They are set out as six papers with obstetric and gynaecological questions mixed. We have tried to cover all the main topics and apologize for any omissions. Answers are provided at the back of the book (true answers only – in bold print) with brief explanations for the false answers. The reader is referred to the appropriate topics in *Key Topics in Obstetrics and Gynaecology* for further information. If that information is not available or supplementary reading is advised, references have been added.

We have tried to ensure that the questions are accurate and unambiguous. Sometimes the more knowledge you obtain the more difficult it becomes to answer a question. Read the questions carefully but do not look for the hidden meanings – there are none. We take responsibility for all of the views expressed. By use of extensive references we hope to show you why we have decided on each answer. You may disagree with some of our thoughts, if so please write (or email) the publishers and let us know. The idea of these questions are to familiarize yourselves with the examination format, to stimulate thought and encourage you to read in greater depth those areas where you are uncertain.

We would like to thank Charlotte, Tini and Gitasri for putting up with us over the last 6 months. We would like to thank Jonathan Ray at BIOS for his encouragement and Mr Roger Jackson, the Examination Secretary at the Royal College of Obstetricians and Gynaecologists for allowing us to reproduce the answer sheet.

Finally, for those amongst you of nervous disposition, the only true answer for the specimen statements on induction of labour is number 4, the others are false. (*Reference*: Induction of labour. RCOG Guideline 16, July 1998). Good luck.

Andrew Pickersgill
Apollo Meskhi
Sudipta Paul

Royal College of Obstetricians and Gynaecologists
Part 2 Membership Examination

Surname (Family Name)

Other Name(s)

T=True

F=False

Candidate Number

c0ɔ	c0ɔ	c0ɔ	c0ɔ
c1ɔ	c1ɔ	c1ɔ	c1ɔ
c2ɔ	c2ɔ	c2ɔ	c2ɔ
c3ɔ	c3ɔ	c3ɔ	c3ɔ
c4ɔ	c4ɔ	c4ɔ	c4ɔ
c5ɔ	c5ɔ	c5ɔ	c5ɔ
c6ɔ	c6ɔ	c6ɔ	c6ɔ
c7ɔ	c7ɔ	c7ɔ	c7ɔ
c8ɔ	c8ɔ	c8ɔ	c8ɔ
c9ɔ	c9ɔ	c9ɔ	c9ɔ

IMPORTANT - When you have finished, check that you have answered EVERY question either true or false.
If you leave any question blank it will be scored the same as an incorrect answer.

1 cTɔ cFɔ	31 cTɔ cFɔ	61 cTɔ cFɔ	91 cTɔ cFɔ	121 cTɔ cFɔ
2 cTɔ cFɔ	32 cTɔ cFɔ	62 cTɔ cFɔ	92 cTɔ cFɔ	122 cTɔ cFɔ
3 cTɔ cFɔ	33 cTɔ cFɔ	63 cTɔ cFɔ	93 cTɔ cFɔ	123 cTɔ cFɔ
4 cTɔ cFɔ	34 cTɔ cFɔ	64 cTɔ cFɔ	94 cTɔ cFɔ	124 cTɔ cFɔ
5 cTɔ cFɔ	35 cTɔ cFɔ	65 cTɔ cFɔ	95 cTɔ cFɔ	125 cTɔ cFɔ
6 cTɔ cFɔ	36 cTɔ cFɔ	66 cTɔ cFɔ	96 cTɔ cFɔ	126 cTɔ cFɔ
7 cTɔ cFɔ	37 cTɔ cFɔ	67 cTɔ cFɔ	97 cTɔ cFɔ	127 cTɔ cFɔ
8 cTɔ cFɔ	38 cTɔ cFɔ	68 cTɔ cFɔ	98 cTɔ cFɔ	128 cTɔ cFɔ
9 cTɔ cFɔ	39 cTɔ cFɔ	69 cTɔ cFɔ	99 cTɔ cFɔ	129 cTɔ cFɔ
10 cTɔ cFɔ	40 cTɔ cFɔ	70 cTɔ cFɔ	100 cTɔ cFɔ	130 cTɔ cFɔ
11 cTɔ cFɔ	41 cTɔ cFɔ	71 cTɔ cFɔ	101 cTɔ cFɔ	131 cTɔ cFɔ
12 cTɔ cFɔ	42 cTɔ cFɔ	72 cTɔ cFɔ	102 cTɔ cFɔ	132 cTɔ cFɔ
13 cTɔ cFɔ	43 cTɔ cFɔ	73 cTɔ cFɔ	103 cTɔ cFɔ	133 cTɔ cFɔ
14 cTɔ cFɔ	44 cTɔ cFɔ	74 cTɔ cFɔ	104 cTɔ cFɔ	134 cTɔ cFɔ
15 cTɔ cFɔ	45 cTɔ cFɔ	75 cTɔ cFɔ	105 cTɔ cFɔ	135 cTɔ cFɔ
16 cTɔ cFɔ	46 cTɔ cFɔ	76 cTɔ cFɔ	106 cTɔ cFɔ	136 cTɔ cFɔ
17 cTɔ cFɔ	47 cTɔ cFɔ	77 cTɔ cFɔ	107 cTɔ cFɔ	137 cTɔ cFɔ
18 cTɔ cFɔ	48 cTɔ cFɔ	78 cTɔ cFɔ	108 cTɔ cFɔ	138 cTɔ cFɔ
19 cTɔ cFɔ	49 cTɔ cFɔ	79 cTɔ cFɔ	109 cTɔ cFɔ	139 cTɔ cFɔ
20 cTɔ cFɔ	50 cTɔ cFɔ	80 cTɔ cFɔ	110 cTɔ cFɔ	140 cTɔ cFɔ
21 cTɔ cFɔ	51 cTɔ cFɔ	81 cTɔ cFɔ	111 cTɔ cFɔ	141 cTɔ cFɔ
22 cTɔ cFɔ	52 cTɔ cFɔ	82 cTɔ cFɔ	112 cTɔ cFɔ	142 cTɔ cFɔ
23 cTɔ cFɔ	53 cTɔ cFɔ	83 cTɔ cFɔ	113 cTɔ cFɔ	143 cTɔ cFɔ
24 cTɔ cFɔ	54 cTɔ cFɔ	84 cTɔ cFɔ	114 cTɔ cFɔ	144 cTɔ cFɔ
25 cTɔ cFɔ	55 cTɔ cFɔ	85 cTɔ cFɔ	115 cTɔ cFɔ	145 cTɔ cFɔ
26 cTɔ cFɔ	56 cTɔ cFɔ	86 cTɔ cFɔ	116 cTɔ cFɔ	146 cTɔ cFɔ
27 cTɔ cFɔ	57 cTɔ cFɔ	87 cTɔ cFɔ	117 cTɔ cFɔ	147 cTɔ cFɔ
28 cTɔ cFɔ	58 cTɔ cFɔ	88 cTɔ cFɔ	118 cTɔ cFɔ	148 cTɔ cFɔ
29 cTɔ cFɔ	59 cTɔ cFɔ	89 cTɔ cFɔ	119 cTɔ cFɔ	149 cTɔ cFɔ
30 cTɔ cFɔ	60 cTɔ cFɔ	90 cTɔ cFɔ	120 cTɔ cFɔ	150 cTɔ cFɔ

Check that you have answered every question either True or False.

This form will be read by a machine
Please use the HB pencil provided
Mark each answer with a single horizontal line   ⊏T⊐   ⊏F⊐
If you make a mistake erase it completely
Do NOT mark with ticks, crosses or circles
Do not forget to enter your name and candidate number properly

T=True

F=False

IMPORTANT - When you have finished, check that you have answered EVERY question either true or false.
If you leave any question blank it will be scored the same as an incorrect answer.

151 ⊏T⊐ ⊏F⊐	181 ⊏T⊐ ⊏F⊐	211 ⊏T⊐ ⊏F⊐	241 ⊏T⊐ ⊏F⊐	271 ⊏T⊐ ⊏F⊐
152 ⊏T⊐ ⊏F⊐	182 ⊏T⊐ ⊏F⊐	212 ⊏T⊐ ⊏F⊐	242 ⊏T⊐ ⊏F⊐	272 ⊏T⊐ ⊏F⊐
153 ⊏T⊐ ⊏F⊐	183 ⊏T⊐ ⊏F⊐	213 ⊏T⊐ ⊏F⊐	243 ⊏T⊐ ⊏F⊐	273 ⊏T⊐ ⊏F⊐
154 ⊏T⊐ ⊏F⊐	184 ⊏T⊐ ⊏F⊐	214 ⊏T⊐ ⊏F⊐	244 ⊏T⊐ ⊏F⊐	274 ⊏T⊐ ⊏F⊐
155 ⊏T⊐ ⊏F⊐	185 ⊏T⊐ ⊏F⊐	215 ⊏T⊐ ⊏F⊐	245 ⊏T⊐ ⊏F⊐	275 ⊏T⊐ ⊏F⊐
156 ⊏T⊐ ⊏F⊐	186 ⊏T⊐ ⊏F⊐	216 ⊏T⊐ ⊏F⊐	246 ⊏T⊐ ⊏F⊐	276 ⊏T⊐ ⊏F⊐
157 ⊏T⊐ ⊏F⊐	187 ⊏T⊐ ⊏F⊐	217 ⊏T⊐ ⊏F⊐	247 ⊏T⊐ ⊏F⊐	277 ⊏T⊐ ⊏F⊐
158 ⊏T⊐ ⊏F⊐	188 ⊏T⊐ ⊏F⊐	218 ⊏T⊐ ⊏F⊐	248 ⊏T⊐ ⊏F⊐	278 ⊏T⊐ ⊏F⊐
159 ⊏T⊐ ⊏F⊐	189 ⊏T⊐ ⊏F⊐	219 ⊏T⊐ ⊏F⊐	249 ⊏T⊐ ⊏F⊐	279 ⊏T⊐ ⊏F⊐
160 ⊏T⊐ ⊏F⊐	190 ⊏T⊐ ⊏F⊐	220 ⊏T⊐ ⊏F⊐	250 ⊏T⊐ ⊏F⊐	280 ⊏T⊐ ⊏F⊐
161 ⊏T⊐ ⊏F⊐	191 ⊏T⊐ ⊏F⊐	221 ⊏T⊐ ⊏F⊐	251 ⊏T⊐ ⊏F⊐	281 ⊏T⊐ ⊏F⊐
162 ⊏T⊐ ⊏F⊐	192 ⊏T⊐ ⊏F⊐	222 ⊏T⊐ ⊏F⊐	252 ⊏T⊐ ⊏F⊐	282 ⊏T⊐ ⊏F⊐
163 ⊏T⊐ ⊏F⊐	193 ⊏T⊐ ⊏F⊐	223 ⊏T⊐ ⊏F⊐	253 ⊏T⊐ ⊏F⊐	283 ⊏T⊐ ⊏F⊐
164 ⊏T⊐ ⊏F⊐	194 ⊏T⊐ ⊏F⊐	224 ⊏T⊐ ⊏F⊐	254 ⊏T⊐ ⊏F⊐	284 ⊏T⊐ ⊏F⊐
165 ⊏T⊐ ⊏F⊐	195 ⊏T⊐ ⊏F⊐	225 ⊏T⊐ ⊏F⊐	255 ⊏T⊐ ⊏F⊐	285 ⊏T⊐ ⊏F⊐
166 ⊏T⊐ ⊏F⊐	196 ⊏T⊐ ⊏F⊐	226 ⊏T⊐ ⊏F⊐	256 ⊏T⊐ ⊏F⊐	286 ⊏T⊐ ⊏F⊐
167 ⊏T⊐ ⊏F⊐	197 ⊏T⊐ ⊏F⊐	227 ⊏T⊐ ⊏F⊐	257 ⊏T⊐ ⊏F⊐	287 ⊏T⊐ ⊏F⊐
168 ⊏T⊐ ⊏F⊐	198 ⊏T⊐ ⊏F⊐	228 ⊏T⊐ ⊏F⊐	258 ⊏T⊐ ⊏F⊐	288 ⊏T⊐ ⊏F⊐
169 ⊏T⊐ ⊏F⊐	199 ⊏T⊐ ⊏F⊐	229 ⊏T⊐ ⊏F⊐	259 ⊏T⊐ ⊏F⊐	289 ⊏T⊐ ⊏F⊐
170 ⊏T⊐ ⊏F⊐	200 ⊏T⊐ ⊏F⊐	230 ⊏T⊐ ⊏F⊐	260 ⊏T⊐ ⊏F⊐	290 ⊏T⊐ ⊏F⊐
171 ⊏T⊐ ⊏F⊐	201 ⊏T⊐ ⊏F⊐	231 ⊏T⊐ ⊏F⊐	261 ⊏T⊐ ⊏F⊐	291 ⊏T⊐ ⊏F⊐
172 ⊏T⊐ ⊏F⊐	202 ⊏T⊐ ⊏F⊐	232 ⊏T⊐ ⊏F⊐	262 ⊏T⊐ ⊏F⊐	292 ⊏T⊐ ⊏F⊐
173 ⊏T⊐ ⊏F⊐	203 ⊏T⊐ ⊏F⊐	233 ⊏T⊐ ⊏F⊐	263 ⊏T⊐ ⊏F⊐	293 ⊏T⊐ ⊏F⊐
174 ⊏T⊐ ⊏F⊐	204 ⊏T⊐ ⊏F⊐	234 ⊏T⊐ ⊏F⊐	264 ⊏T⊐ ⊏F⊐	294 ⊏T⊐ ⊏F⊐
175 ⊏T⊐ ⊏F⊐	205 ⊏T⊐ ⊏F⊐	235 ⊏T⊐ ⊏F⊐	265 ⊏T⊐ ⊏F⊐	295 ⊏T⊐ ⊏F⊐
176 ⊏T⊐ ⊏F⊐	206 ⊏T⊐ ⊏F⊐	236 ⊏T⊐ ⊏F⊐	266 ⊏T⊐ ⊏F⊐	296 ⊏T⊐ ⊏F⊐
177 ⊏T⊐ ⊏F⊐	207 ⊏T⊐ ⊏F⊐	237 ⊏T⊐ ⊏F⊐	267 ⊏T⊐ ⊏F⊐	297 ⊏T⊐ ⊏F⊐
178 ⊏T⊐ ⊏F⊐	208 ⊏T⊐ ⊏F⊐	238 ⊏T⊐ ⊏F⊐	268 ⊏T⊐ ⊏F⊐	298 ⊏T⊐ ⊏F⊐
179 ⊏T⊐ ⊏F⊐	209 ⊏T⊐ ⊏F⊐	239 ⊏T⊐ ⊏F⊐	269 ⊏T⊐ ⊏F⊐	299 ⊏T⊐ ⊏F⊐
180 ⊏T⊐ ⊏F⊐	210 ⊏T⊐ ⊏F⊐	240 ⊏T⊐ ⊏F⊐	270 ⊏T⊐ ⊏F⊐	300 ⊏T⊐ ⊏F⊐

Check that you have answered every question either True or False.

System Design by Speedwell Computing Services. 01604 410041   Mark Reflex® by NCS: NM-01317.654321 1-D3803 Printed in the U.K.

PAPER ONE

Allow 2 hours for completion of this paper

Regarding early pregnancy loss

1. A woman presents for the second time with vaginal bleeding and lower abdominal pain, her cervix is closed. A scan 1 week previously noted an intrauterine gestation sac. On rescanning she is now found to have an empty uterus. She can be reassurred that she has suffered a complete miscarriage and needs no follow up
2. A woman presenting in early pregnancy with heavy vaginal bleeding, an open cervical os and an echogenic area in the uterine cavity should be told that she is having an inevitable abortion and needs an immediate uterine evacuation
3. An incomplete miscarriage differs from a complete miscarriage as judged by a closed cervical os in presence of heavy vaginal bleeding
4. A Rhesus negative woman presents with a complete miscarriage, the injection of anti-D is unnecessary
5. In a woman with a threatened miscarriage, if a scan shows a fetal heart the risk of a miscarriage is 30%

Raised maternal serum alpha-fetoprotein (MSAFP) concentrations are associated with the following fetal abnormalities

6. Polycystic kidney
7. Closed spina bifida
8. Gastroschisis
9. Congenital nephrosis (Finnish type)
10. Epidermolysis bullosa
11. Tay–Sach's disease
12. Teratoma
13. Duodenal atresia

Impotence may be caused by

14. Sulphasalazine therapy
15. Chronic renal failure

Recognized causes of non-immune hydrops fetalis include

16. Renal agenesis
17. Duodenal atresia
18. Cystic adenomatous malformation
19. Cytomegalovirus infection

In a paper describing the use of a new drug for the treatment of hypertension in pregnancy you read: 'The mean fall in diastolic blood pressure in the treated group (n = 30) was 10 mmHg +/-3 (SD) and in the control group (n = 29) given placebo the mean fall was 4 mmHg +/-2.6 (SD). Using the t-test, p>0.001.' The following statements are correct:

20. Assuming a normal distribution, approximately 68% of the treated group would have shown a fall in the diastolic pressure of between 7 and 13 mmHg
21. The difference observed in the fall of blood pressure between the two groups did not reach a level of statistical significance
22. If the trial was properly conducted, the doctors involved should have known which patients were receiving the active drug and which the placebo
23. The most appropriate way to allocate patients to the drug and to the placebo group would have been to give the drug or placebo to alternate patients
24. It would be possible to calculate the value of χ (Chi-squared) on the data given

With regard to hysterectomy

25. One in ten women in the UK will have a hysterectomy before becoming menopausal
26. Vaginal hysterectomy is performed four times more rarely than abdominal
27. Overall mortality is 4.1–14.6/10 000 hysterectomies
28. Overall morbidity is 500–1000/10 000 hysterectomies
29. Vault prolapse is a common complication of vaginal hysterectomy and can be prevented by suturing the utero-sacral ligaments together
30. 30–40% of ovaries can be removed vaginally if desired
31. Vaginal hysterectomy is associated with an overall complication rate 40–50% less than for abdominal hysterectomy

The following drugs administered in pregnancy may have adverse effects on the newborn

32. Betablockers
33. Barbiturates
34. Magnesium sulphate
35. Naloxone hydrochloride

In the UK the following incidences are correct

36. Toxoplasmosis   2/1000
37. Down's syndrome   1.3/1000
38. Rhesus sensitization   15/1000

The following are not advantages of magnetic resonance imaging (MRI) in investigating cervical tumours

39. It is safe
40. It can be used in pregnancy
41. MRI demonstrates depth of stromal invasion (in up to 90% of cases)
42. It may show total tumour volume
43. MRI is superior to clinical staging and CT images

Ovarian cysts are relative contraindications to the use of

44. The combined pill
45. Depo-provera
46. Norplant

Prostaglandins

47. Are polypeptides
48. Hypertonus cannot be reversed by beta-mimetics
49. $PGF_{2\alpha}$ is 20 times more potent than PGE_2 in causing uterine contractions
50. PGE_2 is five times more potent than $PGF_{2\alpha}$ in ripening the cervix
51. $PGF_{2\alpha}$ is commonly used in induction of labour
52. PGE_2 is the drug of choice in refractory post-partum haemorrhage at Caesarean section
53. Are diuretics

Regarding the progesterone only pill (POP)

54. 60% of women using it will ovulate
55. Ideally it should be taken just before bedtime
56. The Pearl Index is higher in the older reproductive age group
57. It is associated with a higher risk of an ectopic pregnancy than for a non-user
58. It is at least as effective as the combined contraceptive pill
59. Amenorrhoea/oligomenorrhoea occurs in 10–20%
60. It is contraindicated in lactating mothers with benign breast disease
61. It is not contraindicated in latent diabetes mellitus
62. It contains norethisterone and is taken from day 5 of the menstrual cycle for 21 days followed by a 7-day break
63. It should always be taken within $+/-3$ hours of the usual taking time to achieve reliable contraceptive efficacy
64. Liver enzyme inducers reduce its efficacy

The following conditions may deteriorate during pregnancy

65. Sarcoidosis
66. Systemic lupus erythematosus (SLE)
67. Coeliac disease
68. von Willebrand's disease
69. Crohn's disease

Psychiatric disorders of childbirth

70. Postnatal mental disorder is less likely to be a serious illness than one not associated with childbirth
71. Being single, ambivalent about the pregnancy and undergoing antenatal hospital admissions are all risk factors for postnatal depression
72. For a well woman with a family history of a serious affective disorder, the risk of postnatal depression is higher than that for a woman with a history of postnatal depression
73. Among women with puerperal affective disorder, two-thirds have the manic form
74. Treatment with steroids is highly effective
75. Maternity blues affect up to 30% of all newly confined women

In a 26-year-old woman the serum follicle-stimulating hormone (FSH) concentration may be raised in association with

76. Acromegaly
77. Polycystic ovarian disease
78. Hydatidiform mole
79. Ovarian agenesis
80. Sheehan's syndrome
81. GnRH administration

The following diseases are inherited as autosomal recessive traits

82. Congenital spherocytosis
83. Myotonic dystrophy
84. Nephrogenic diabetes insipidus
85. Congenital heart disease
86. Alkaptonuria

Following a hip fracture, bone densitometry in a 60-year-old woman who is 10 years post-menopausal reveals osteoporosis of the spine and both hips

87. Her bone density will not be improved by prescribing her oestrogen containing HRT
88. If given oestrogens, these will act uniformly at both sites to improve her osteoporosis
89. Sodium etidronate will reduce the risk of further fractures

Management of abnormal smears

90. A third of woman with a single smear showing mild dyskaryosis have CIN 3
91. The risk of invasive malignancy remains equal to that of normal population in women who have undergone excisional treatment for CIN 3
92. Following a hysterectomy for the surgical treatment of CIN 3 annual smears are required for the next 5 years if the CIN was completely removed

Lichen sclerosus

93. Manifests itself with pruritus
94. Histological features include atrophic thinning of the epidermis and loss of rete ridges
95. Is a premalignant condition characterized by cellular atypia
96. Is a condition specific to vulval skin
97. Surgery is the main treatment modality in modern management
98. Progression to invasive carcinoma of the vulva is more likely to occur if lichen sclerosus is associated with squamous cell hyperplasia

Endometrial cancer

99. Constitutes 25–30% of all gynaecological malignancies
100. The commonest type is adenosqamous
101. Pelvic nodes are involved in 5% of poorly differentiated cases
102. Adenosquamous carcinoma has a better prognosis than adenocarcinoma
103. Has a greater tendency to metastasize if it involves the lower uterus rather than the fundus

Regarding syphilis

104. This is the commonest cause of painless genital ulcers
105. Syphilis can be transferred to the fetus transplacentally in early pregnancy
106. VDRL detects antibodies to treponemal cardiolipin antigen
107. VDRL is a highly specific test for the diagnosis of syphilis
108. A positive VDRL could be a manifestation of SLE
109. Fluorescent treponemal antibody (FTA) test has specificity similar to VDRL
110. Dark ground microscopy for the diagnosis of syphilis has been abandoned
111. Neonatal syphilis syndrome occurs due to transmission of the infection to the fetus after 5 months' gestation
112. The patient should be regarded as being infectious for up to 2 years
113. Primary syphilis is associated with a generalized rash
114. Syphilis may cause Horner's syndrome

Trigger events that could initiate a risk management protocol include

115. Birth of a baby with a structural abnormality
116. Admission to SCBU
117. Failed trial of instrumental delivery
118. Failed termination of pregnancy
119. Peritonitis after laparoscopy
120. Failed instrumental delivery

Termination of pregnancy

121. Is associated with an increased risk of recurrent miscarriage
122. Is associated with an increased risk of pelvic pain

Sarcoma botryoides

123. Is a tumour of teenage years
124. Occurs in association with *in utero* exposure to synthetic oestrogens
125. The treatment of choice is combination chemotherapy

Premenstrual syndrome

126. Is a rare condition
127. Is diagnosed by retrospective symptom charts
128. Hormonal imbalance is a proven underlying cause

Syntocinon augmentation of labour

129. May cause or aggravate neonatal jaundice
130. Is more often required in multiparous women
131. May have to be reduced as labour progresses

Factors predisposing to genuine stress incontinence (GSI) include

132. Multiple Caesarean deliveries
133. Chronic constipation
134. Chronic bronchitis
135. Oestrogen deficiency
136. Gross obesity

In treating preterm labour with ritodrine, certain caution should be taken with

137. Adrenergic stimulants
138. Tricyclic antidepressants
139. Thiazide diuretics
140. Twins
141. Aortic stenosis
142. Transverse lie

Endometrial cystic glandular hyperplasia

143. Occurs with ovulatory failure
144. May predispose to endometrial carcinoma
145. Is associated with low oestrogen levels
146. Is transmitted by a virus in cheese
147. Generally occurs post-menopausally

Thyrotoxicosis in pregnancy

148. Subtotal thyroidectomy is 'safe' during the first trimester
149. Propyl-thiouracil should be stopped 6 weeks prior to delivery
150. Over-treatment with carbimazole may cause fetal goitre
151. Measurement of T4 is helpful in monitoring the disease process
152. The disease deteriorates in pregnancy
153. Mild disease may not be distinguishable from normal changes of pregnancy in mid-trimester
154. An anti-thyroid drug and thyroxine is the optimum treatment
155. Propranolol should be added from 36 weeks onwards

Group B streptococcal infections

156. Is the commonest cause of non-iatrogenic bacterial sepsis
157. 20–25% of women are carriers
158. Mortality rates are 20% in affected neonates
159. Infections can be eliminated by screening all women at 28 weeks
160. Risk factors include preterm labour, ruptured membranes of greater than 18 hours and intra-partum fever.

There is a recognized association between gynaecomastia and

161. Carcinoma of the stomach
162. Normal puberty
163. Hyperprolactinaemia
164. Carcinoid tumour
165. Cirrhosis of the liver
166. Klinefelter's syndrome
167. 5-alpha reductase deficiency
168. Spironolactone
169. Phaeochromocytoma

Asymptomatic bacteriuria

170. Is found in 2% of pregnant women
171. Is associated with an increase in perinatal mortality
172. Predisposes to acute pyelonephritis
173. Is defined as a bacterial count of greater than 10 000 organisms/ml
174. Should be checked for at each antenatal visit
175. Predisposes to glomerulonephritis
176. Predisposes to hypertension
177. Requires an IVP after pregnancy
178. Causes anaemia
179. Causes neonatal death
180. Causes preterm labour

Eclampsia

181. Less than 10% of cases occur during the post-partum period
182. Has a poorer prognosis if it occurs ante-partum than during the intra-partum period
183. Hydralazine treatment is contraindicated with chlormethiazole
184. Cerebral haemorrhage is the commonest cause of death
185. Diuresis is a prodromal symptom prior to a fit
186. Peripheral oedema is common
187. The circulating blood volume is increased
188. Immediate delivery under general anaesthesia is the management of choice
189. Oxprenolol 160 mg per day would be the best antihypertensive therapy
190. Delivery is contraindicated before 28 weeks gestation
191. Renal failure is the commonest cause of death

GnRH agonists are used effectively in the treatment of

192. Leiomyosarcomas
193. Premenstrual tension
194. Adenomyosis
195. Menstrual migraines
196. Hidradenitis suppurativa
197. Precocious puberty

Maternal cardiovascular system (CVS) in pregnancy

198. The majority of heart murmurs detected for the first time during pregnancy are due to functional mitral regurgitation
199. Anticoagulants administered to patients with heart valve prostheses should be withdrawn at 36 weeks gestation
200. In patients with uncorrected chronic rheumatic valvular heart disease, crystalline penicillin alone provides adequate prophylaxis at the time of delivery
201. Supraventricular arrhythmias occur with greater frequency than in a non-pregnant woman
202. Frusemide is contraindicated for the treatment of heart failure

The following are true when comparing modern obstetric practices regarding instrumental deliveries

203. Forceps can be used if the cervix is not fully dilated, a ventouse cannot
204. Forceps are associated with a twofold increase in trauma to the birth canal, but a twofold decrease in cephalohaematomas when compared to a ventouse
205. Forceps double the risk of anal sphincter damage and bowel symptoms compared to ventouse

Vaginal pH

206. During reproductive life it is lowest during menstruation
207. Rises post-menopausally
208. Declines from birth through the first years of life
209. Low vaginal pH is caused by cervical secretions
210. High pH predisposes to vaginal infections
211. Atrophic vaginitis is associated with a high pH
212. Oestrogen replacement therapy increases vaginal pH

Predisposing factors to face presentation include

213. Iniencephaly
214. Multiple pregnancy
215. Placenta praevia
216. Increasing maternal age
217. Multiparity
218. Prematurity
219. Polyhydramnios
220. Bicornuate uterus

The following are not associated with hirsutism

221. Anorexia nervosa
222. Hyperthecosis of the ovary
223. Testicular feminization
224. Acromegaly
225. Juvenile hypothyroidism
226. Hilar cell tumour

Ovarian tumours may be associated with

227. Peutz–Jegher syndrome
228. Gorlin's syndrome
229. Gonadal dysgenesis
230. Kallman's syndrome

In massive obstetric haemorrhage

231. Platelets should be given early
232. Fresh frozen plasma should be given early
233. Colloids are preferable to crystalloids
234. 10% calcium chloride should be given routinely

Progestogens, when given with oestrogens to post-menopausal women

235. Decrease LDL cholesterol
236. Cause endometrial hyperplasia
237. Protect the patient from developing breast cancer
238. May cause depression
239. Act as insulin antagonists
240. Protect against bone loss

Deep venous thrombosis (DVT) and pregnancy

241. 80% of DVTs occur in the right leg
242. Clinical examination misses 50%
243. Treatment should be commenced on clinical grounds if the confirmatory tests are not immediately available
244. The risk of pulmonary embolism in patients with DVT is 2–5%
245. Occurs primary to pulmonary embolism

Recognized features of Turner's syndrome include

246. Recurrent miscarriage
247. Elevated serum gonadotrophin levels
248. Renal abnormalities
249. Coarctation of the aorta
250. Red–green colour blindness
251. Chromatin positive buccal cells
252. Anosmia
253. Bone age appropriate for age

The menstrual cycle

254. New endometrial growth begins during menstruation
255. In irregular cycles the luteal phase is always constant (14 days) whereas the follicular phase alters
256. Ovulation coincides with the LH peak
257. A normal day 21 progesterone is a direct indicator of ovulation
258. Menstruation occurs following oestrogen withdrawal
259. The average size of a follicle at the time of ovulation is 23 mm
260. GnRH pulses increase in frequency and amplitude throughout the follicular phase
261. Thecal cells of the ovarian stroma exclusively secrete androstenedione

Intrauterine contraceptive devices (IUCD)

262. All types are contraindications to MRI scan
263. Increase the risk of preterm delivery
264. Induces a foreign body reaction in the endometrium which interferes with blastocyst implantation
265. If inserted into the uterus after the age of 40 can be left *in situ* indefinitely
266. Are recommended for renal transplant receipients
267. The risk of ascending infection into the uterine cavity is the highest during the first 2–3 weeks after insertion
268. Contraceptive efficacy of copper devices is proportional to the weight of the copper loaded on the device
269. Protects from ectopic pregnancies as effectively as from intrauterine pregnancies
270. Most modern IUCDS are effective for 5 years after insertion
271. The commonest reasons for removal are bleeding and pain

In rupture of the uterus, the following may occur

272. Hypotension
273. Increased uterine contractions
274. Haematuria
275. Vaginal bleeding
276. Fetal distress

Causes of pruritus ani include

277. Anal fissure
278. Diverticulitis coli
279. Rectal prolapse
280. *Ascaris lumbricoides* infestation
281. Perianal condylomata

SLE in pregnancy

282. There is a high risk of puerperal exacerbation
283. Increases the risk of spontaneous miscarriage
284. Is associated with symptoms similar to pre-eclampsia
285. Should never be treated with azathioprine
286. The presence of lupus anticoagulant decreases the risk of thrombosis

The following conditions can be detected by ultrasound scanning of the fetus

287. Duodenal atresia
288. Syndactyly
289. Hydrops fetalis
290. Fetal polycystic kidneys
291. Congenital heart block

Regarding puberty

292. Puberty is associated with nocturnal pulses of LH occurring during REM sleep
293. Peak height velocity appears after menarche
294. Puberty occurs at the average age of 11 in the UK

Regarding dural tap

295. The incidence is 1–2%
296. The incidence is operator-dependant
297. It has neurological implications
298. Post-dural puncture headaches commonly occur immediately with the puncture
299. It may be followed by headache in 70% of cases
300. A blood patch takes effect within 2–3 days

ANSWERS TO PAPER ONE

The numbers of the correct answers are given

Regarding early pregnancy loss
(Abortion spontaneous/recurrent)
With the first two scenarios you cannot rule out an ectopic pregnancy. Unless a woman is haemodynamically compromised inevitable abortions can be managed conservatively. The cervical os is open with an incomplete miscarriage. The type of miscarriage is not important, all Rhesus-negative women who have suffered the loss of a pregnancy require anti-D. The risk of fetal loss is less than 5% after visualization of a fetal heartbeat.

Raised MSAFP are associated with the following fetal abnormalities
6, 8, 9, 10, 11, 12, 13   (Prenatal diagnosis)
MSAFP is raised in open spina bifida and other neural tube defects (anencephaly). Other associations include advanced gestational age (up to 32 weeks), fetal exomphalos, aplasia cutis, obstructive uropathies, congenital cystic adenomatoid malformations, amniotic band disruption, placental and umbilical cord tumours, maternal liver disease, certain chromosomal disorders, preterm labour and IUGR.
MSAFP is not raised if the fetus is affected by cystic fibrosis (but can be if the mother is), Down's syndrome, Duchenne muscular dystrophy, isolated fetal hydrocephaly, congenital adrenal hyperplasia, Potter's syndrome nor in women taking the oral contraceptive pill.

References
Neilson JP. Antenatal diagnosis of fetal abnormality. In: Whitfield CR, ed. *Dewhurst's Textbook of Obstetrics and Gynaecology for Postgraduates*, 5th edn, Oxford: Blackwell Science, 1995; 121–129.
Williamson RA. Abnormalities of alpha-fetoprotein and other biochemical tests. In: James DK, Steer PJ, Weiner CP, Gonik B, eds. *High Risk Pregnancy Management Options*. London: WB Saunders Company, 1994; 643–659.

Impotence may be caused by
15
Sulphasalazine therapy may cause reversible oligozoospermia.

Recognized causes of non-immune hydrops fetalis include

17, 18, 19   (Hydrops fetalis)

Renal agenesis is associated with oligohydramnios. Non-immune hydrops is rare but accounts for 3% of overall perinatal mortality. It is caused by fetal anaemia (e.g. alpha thalassaemia, G-6-PD deficiency), cardiac failure (e.g. fetal tachyarrythmia, congenital heart defects, myocarditis), reduced osmotic pressure (hypoproteinaemia) and space-occupying lesions that obstruct venous return (cystic adenomatous malformation, diaphragmatic hernia). Infective agents may lead to haemolysis and subsequent anaemia (e.g. parvovirus, leptospira). Impaired lymphatic drainage has also been implicated (e.g. cystic hygroma, trisomy 18/21).

Reference

Johnson P, Allan LD and Maxwell DJ. Non-immune hydrops fetalis. In: Studd J, ed. *Progress in Obstetrics and Gynaecology*, Volume 10. Edinburgh: Churchill Livingstone, 1993; 33–50.

Statistical analysis of a new drug for the treatment of hypertension in pregnancy

20, 24

The difference observed in blood pressure fall was statistically significant ($p > 0.001$). In a properly conducted trial (double blind), neither the doctors nor the patients should have known which patients were receiving the active drug and which the placebo. The most appropriate way to allocate patients is to randomize (not to allocate alternately).

Reference

Swinscow TDV, Campbell MJ. *Statistics at Square One*, 8th edn. London: BMJ Publishing Group, 1996; 11–30, 52–85.

With regard to hysterectomy

26, 27, 31   (Abdominal versus vaginal hysterectomy)

One in five women in the UK will have a hysterectomy before becoming menopausal. Overall morbidity is 25–50% (2500–5000/10 000 hysterectomies). Vault prolapse is a relatively uncommon complication of vaginal hysterectomy occurring in 2% which can be prevented by suturing the vault to the uterosacral and cardinal ligaments. Opposing the utero-sacral ligaments reduces the risk of enterocoele formation. 95% of ovaries can be removed vaginally by skilled surgeons.

The following drugs administered in pregnancy may have adverse effects on the newborn

32, 33, 34, 35

Beta blockers may cause neonatal bradycardias and hypoglycaemia. Barbiturates may precipitate withdrawal effects (not normally immediately). Magnesium sulphate like diazepam, diamorphine and pethidine may cause respiratory depression. Naloxone hydrochloride may precipitate withdrawal in babies born to opiate addicts.

Reference

British National Formulary, **35**; March 1998.

In the UK the following incidences are correct
36, 37, 38

The following are not advantages of MRI in investigating cervical tumours
(Radiology)
All false: they are all advantages.

Reference
Carrington BM, Johnson RJ. The role of computed tomography in the investigation of ovarian and cervical cancer. RCOG PACE review 96/04.

Ovarian cysts are relative contraindications to the use of
45, 46
The combined pill reduces the incidence of ovarian cysts. Although progesterone-based contraceptives inhibit ovulation they are associated with the development of functional cysts.

Prostaglandins
50 (Induction of labour, Post-partum haemorrhage)
Prostaglandins are a family of polyunsaturated 20-carbon fatty acids containing a cyclopentane ring and two aliphatic side chains. PGE_2 is five to ten times more potent than $PGF_{2\alpha}$. PGE_2 is used in induction of labour. $PGF_{2\alpha}$ (carboprost tromethamine 250 μg) is the drug of choice in refractory post-partum haemorrhage. Prostaglandins may precipitate pulmonary oedema.

References
Prasad RNV, Adaikan PG. Prostaglandins in obstetrics and gynaecology. In: Ratnam SS, Rao KB and Arulkumaran S, eds. *Obstetrics and Gynaecology for Postgraduates*, Volume I. Hyderabad (India): Orient Longman, 1992; 151–173.
Keirse MJNC. Therapeutic uses of prostaglandins. In: Elder MG, ed. *Ballière's Clinical Obstetrics and Gynaecology International Practice and Research – Prostaglandins*, Volume 6. No 4. London: Baillière Tindall, 1992; 787–808.

Regarding the progesterone only pill (POP)
59, 61, 63, 64 (Contraception and sterilization)
Only 40% of women ovulate with it. It should be taken in the early hours of the evening. The Pearl Index is higher in early reproductive life due to higher natural fertility and lower motivation. It is less effective than the combined pill. The POP is taken continuously, recommended for lactating mothers and does not increase the risk of ectopic compared to non-users. If a pregnancy does occur in a woman using a progestogen-only contraceptive, it is more likely to be an ectopic.

Reference
Webb A. The progesterone only pill. In: *Contraception.* (Update Postgraduate Centre Series), Reed Healthcare Communications, 1995; 16–19.

The following conditions may deteriorate during pregnancy
66, 67
Sarcoidosis is unaffected or improves. SLE may also improve or remain unaffected. Von Willebrand's disease improves and Crohn's disease remains the same.

Psychiatric disorders of childbirth
70, 71   (Puerperal psychosis)
The risk of postnatal depression is increased in women with a family history of a serious affective disorder and a history of postnatal depression, but the risk with the second is higher. Among women with puerperal affective disorder a third are manic and two-thirds are depressive. The role of steroid therapy is not clear. Maternity blues affect 60–70% of newly confined women.

References
Oats M. Psychiatric disorder and childbirth. *Current Obstetrics and Gynaecology*, 1995;_5: 64–69.
Henshaw CA, Cox JL. Postnatal depression. *Current Obstetrics and Gynaecology*, 1995; **5**: 70–74.

In a 26-year-old woman the serum FSH concentration may be raised in association with
79, 81
Acromegaly can be associated with hyperprolactinaemia which reduces GnRH pulsatility and therefore FSH would be low. With polycystic ovarian disease LH is raised. HCG is raised with a hydatidiform mole. Sheehan's syndrome is caused by post-partum pituitary necrosis and therefore is associated with low FSH and LH levels.

The following diseases are inherited as autosomal recessive traits
86
Congenital spherocytosis and myotonic dystrophy are autosomal dominant as are Huntington's chorea, neurofibromatosis, achondroplasia, von Willebrand's disease, tuberous sclerosis, polyposis coli, familial hypercholesterolaemia, adult polycystic kidney disease, multiple exostosis, etc. Congenital heart disease (like neural tube defects, cleft lip and palate and hydrocephaly) has multifactorial inheritance. Nephrogenic diabetes insipidus is X-linked as are red–green colour blindness (8/100 males in UK), fragile X syndrome, pseudohypertrophic Duchenne muscular dystrophy, Becker muscular dystrophy, haemophilia A (factor VIII), haemophilia B (factor IX), glucose-6-phosphate dehydrogenase deficiency, ichthyosis, etc.
Other autosomal recessive conditions are cystic fibrosis, phenylketonuria, glycogen storage disease (von Gierke's disease), adrenogenital syndrome, Tay–Sach's disease, Gaucher disease, thalassaemia and sickle cell disease.

Reference
Connor M and Ferguson-Smith M. *Medical Genetics*, 5th edn Oxford: Blackwell Science, 1997; 69–81.

Hip fracture and osteoporosis

89 (Hormone replacement therapy)

Her bone density will be significantly improved by prescribing her oestrogen containing HRT. Oestrogens do not act uniformly, they have more effect on trabecular (vertebrae) than cortical (appendicular skeleton) bone.

Management of abnormal smears

90 (Premalignant disease of the cervix)

Almost a third of woman with mild cytological abnormalities have grade 3 CIN. In women who have undergone excisional or destructive treatment for CIN 3, the risk of developing an invasive malignancy is five times greater than in the general population. Following a hysterectomy, if the CIN was completely removed, only one vault smear is advised after a year. Annual smears for 5 years are advisable for the follow up of CIN treated with ablative or destructive techniques.

References

Hammond R. Management of women with smears showing mild dyskaryosis. *BMJ*, 1994; **308**: 1383–1384.

Jones MH. The management of the mildly dyskaryotic smear. *British Journal of Obstetrics and Gynaecology*, 1994; **101**: 474–476.

Ten guidelines on cervical smears and colposcopy. Based on *National Co-ordinating Workshop Guideline 1992* and the *Report of the Intercollegiate Working Party 1987.*

Lichen sclerosus

94, 98 (Vulva)

Lichen sclerosus has malignant potential of 0–10%. Cellular atypia is not a feature and it can occur anywhere on the skin, including non-genital areas in 20% of cases. The patient may remain entirely symptom free. The main treatment modality is topical steroid therapy.

References

MacLean AB. Lichen sclerosus. RCOG PACE review 95/09.

Maclean AB. Precursors of vulval cancers. *Current Obstetrics and Gynaecology*, 1993; **3**: 149–156.

MacLean AB. Vulval dystrophy — the passing of a term. *Current Obstetrics and Gynaecology*, 1991; **1**: 97–102.

Endometrial cancer

99, 103 (Uterine tumours)

Adenocarcinoma is the commonest type of endometrial cancer (80% of cases). The commonest sites of spread are the pelvic lymph nodes (iliac and obturator), followed by para-aortic nodes. Inguinal nodes are rarely involved. Pelvic node metastasis are found in up to 26% of poorly differentiated cases and 5.5% of well differentiated cases. The prognosis of adenocarcinoma and adeno-acanthoma are similar and better than that of adenosquamous carcinoma.

References

Lawton FG. Early endometrial carcinoma—no more TAH, BSO and cuff. In: Studd J, ed. *Progress in Obstetrics and Gynaecology*. Volume 10. Edinburgh: Churchill Livingstone, 1993; pp. 403–413.

Irwin CJR. The Management of endometrial carcinoma. *British Journal of Hospital Medicine*, 1996; **55**: 308–309.

Lawton F. The management of endometrial cancer. *British Journal of Obstetrics and Gynaecology*, 1997; **104**: 127–134.

Rose P. Endometrial carcinoma. *The New England Journal of Medicine*, 1996; **335**: 640–648.

Semple D. Endometrial cancer. *British Journal of Hospital Medicine*, 1997; **57**: 260–262.

Regarding syphilis
104, 105, 106, 108, 111, 112, 114   (Sexually transmitted disease)
Syphilis can be transferred to the fetus at any stage during pregnancy or labour. In early pregnancy this is associated with miscarriage and fetal death, in late pregnancy with fetal/neonatal syphilis syndrome. VDRL is the test still widely used. It detects treponemal cardiolipin antigen and has low specificity. It is positive in a number of autoimmune diseases including SLE. The FTA test has higher specificity than VDRL. Dark ground microscopy is used for the diagnosis of primary and early secondary syphilis. A rash is associated with secondary syphilis. Primary syphilis consists of a chancre and local lymphadenopathy.

References

Davey DA, Whitfield CR. Antenatal care in normal pregnancy and pre-pregnant care. In: Whitfield CR, ed. *Dewhurst's Textbook of Obstetrics and Gynaecology for Postgraduates*. 5th edn. Oxford: Blackwell Science, 1995; 109–120.

Stabile I, Chard T, Grudzinskas G. *Clinical Obstetrics and Gynaecology*. New York: Springer-Verlag, 1996; 183–190.

Trigger events that could initiate a risk management protocol include
118, 119, 120   (Risk management)
A trust risk management protocol should be initiated in the case of failed instrumental delivery (not a trial), birth of a baby with undiagnosed structural abnormality, unexpected or late admission of the neonate to the SCBU.

Termination of pregnancy
121, 122 (Therapeutic abortion and the Human Fertilization and Embryology Act 1990)
Recurrent miscarriage is thought to occur due to cervical trauma. Pelvic pain may occur due to complications such as: endometritis, pelvic inflammatory disease and Asherman's syndrome.

Reference

Henshaw RC, Templeton AA. Methods used in first trimester abortion. *Current Obstetrics and Gynaecology*, 1993; **3**: 11–16.

Sarcoma botryoides
125   (Vaginal tumours)
It affects young girls with mean age of 2 years. There is no known association with *in utero* exposure to synthetic oestrogens.

Premenstrual syndrome
(Premenstrual syndrome)
Only 5% of women do not experience symptoms of premenstrual syndrome at all. The diagnosis should be based on the prospective symptom chart. The cause is unknown.

Reference
O'Brian PMS, Abukhalil IEH, Henshaw C. *Current Obstetrics and Gynaecology*, 1995; **5**: 30–35.

Syntocinon augmentation of labour
129, 131   (Induction of labour)
The incidence of neonatal jaundice is increased following the use of syntocinon. It is stated that increased haemolysis is the cause, but it is not clear whether the syntocinon itself or the infusion fluid is responsible for it. As labour progresses the requirement for syntocinon may be reduced in some cases. If the dose of syntocinon is more than optimum, it may cause prolonged hypertonic uterine contraction and fetal distress. IV Terbutaline, SL amylnitrate or GTN spray may be used to relieve hypertonus. Syntocinon is more often required in nulliparous compared to multiparous women.

Reference
Beazley JM. Special Circumstances Affecting Labour. In: Whitfield CR, ed. *Dewhurst's Textbook of Obstetrics and Gynaecology for Postgraduates*, 5th edn. Oxford: Blackwell Science, 1995; 312–332.

Factors predisposing to genuine stress incontinence (GSI) include
133, 134, 135, 136   (Urinary incontinence: urodynamics)
Multiple vaginal deliveries (large babies or with instrumental assistance) are associated with an increased risk of GSI, Caesarean deliveries are not.

References
Cardozo L, Hill S. *Urinary Incontinence*. RCOG PACE review 96/09.
Kelleher CJ, Cardozo LD. The conservative management of female urinary incontinence. In: *The Year Book of The RCOG 1994*; 123–135.
Richmond D. The incontinent women: 1. *British Journal of Hospital Medicine*, 1993; **50**, 418–423.

In treating preterm labour with ritodrine, certain caution should be taken with
137, 138, 139, 140, 141 (Premature labour)
Ritodrine is a beta mimetic drug, which increases the heart rate and plasma glucose concentration. Adrenergic stimulants and tricyclic antidepressants increase the heart rate and may precipitate arrhythmia if used concurrently with ritodrine. Its use is contraindicated in heart disease, thyrotoxicosis, chorioamnionitis etc. It should be used very cautiously in diabetes (thiazide causes hyperglycaemia) and multiple pregnancy. In the 1996 report of the Confidential Enquiry into Maternal Deaths, maternal deaths from pulmonary oedema have been reported following the use of ritodrine. Maintaining a tight fluid balance has been recommended.

References
Beta-agonists for the care of women in preterm labour. *RCOG Guidelines 1a*, 1997.
Report on Confidential Enquiries into Maternal Deaths in the United Kingdom, 1991–1993.
  London: HMSO, 1996.

Endometrial cystic glandular hyperplasia
143, 144 (Uterine tumours)
This generally occurs premenopausally and is associated with raised oestrogen levels and anovulatory conditions (PCO). The risk of progression to cancer is low.

Thyrotoxicosis in pregnancy
150, 153 (Thyroid and pregnancy)
Subtotal thyroidectomy is 'safe' in the second trimester (First trimester–miscarriage, Third trimester–preterm labour). There is no need to stop propyl-thiouracil 6 weeks before delivery, or to add propranolol from 36 weeks. As the T4 level in normal pregnancy increases due to raised thyroid binding globulin level, its measurement is not helpful in monitoring the disease process (free T3, T4 and free thyroxine index are useful). The disease often improves in pregnancy due to immunosuppression because of raised steroid levels. The combination of thyroxine and antithyroid drug is unhelpful, because as the passage of thyroxine through the placenta is negligible, additional thyroxine only increases the requirements for the antithyroid drug. Antithyroid drugs readily cross the placenta and have a suppressive effect on the fetal thyroid gland leading to the formation of a goitre. The optimum treatment is to use the minimum dose of the antithyroid drug necessary to keep the mother euthyroid.

References
Kennedy RL, Darne, EJ. Disorders of the thyroid gland during pregnancy and the
  post-partum period. In: Studd J, ed. *Progress in Obstetrics and Gynaecology*,
  Volume 11. Edinburgh: Churchill Livingstone, 1994; 125–140.
Ramsay I. Thyroid disease. In: De Swiet M, ed. *Medical Disorders in Obstetrics*
  Practice, 2nd edn. Oxford: Blackwell Scientific Publications, 1990; 633–659.

Group B streptococcal infections
156, 157, 158, 160
Screening all women at 28 weeks can reduce infections.

Reference
Van Oppen C, Feldman R. Antibiotic prophylaxis of neonatal group B streptococcal
infections. *BMJ* 1993; **306**: 411–412.

There is a recognized association between gynaecomastia and
161, 162, 163, 165, 166, 167, 168
Gynaecomastia occurs secondary to hypogonadism. This may be acquired (castration,
alcoholism, renal failure) or congenital (Klinefelter's syndrome, 5-alpha reductase
deficiency). Hypogonadism may also occur secondary to hyperprolactinaemia and
reduced gonadotrophins (GnRH therapy, Kallman's syndrome). Pubertal gynaecomastia occurs in about 50% of boys and is usually asymmetrical, resolving within 18
months. Carcinoid tumours secrete serotonin, (oestrogen-secreting tumours of the
testis or adrenal, and HCG-producing tumours of the testis and lung may cause
gynaecomastia). Phaeochromocytomas secrete catecholamines. Other causes are
antiandrogenic drugs (cimetidine, spironolactone, cyproterone) and oestrogenic drugs
(digitalis, cannabis, diamorphine).

References
Drury PL. Endocrinology. In: Kumar PJ, Clark ML. *Clinical Medicine*. London:
Ballière Tindall.
The breast. In: Mann CV, Russell RCG, eds. *Bailey & Love's Short Practice of
Surgery*, 21st edn. London: Chapman & Hall, 1992; 788–821.

Asymptomatic bacteriuria
171, 172, 180   (Renal tract in pregnancy)
It is found in 5% of pregnant women and is defined as a bacterial count of greater
than 100 000 organisms/ml of clean caught mid-stream urine. It predisposes to
pyelonephritis in 30% of cases. There is debate about screening at the booking visit
but it is not indicated at each visit. It should be treated with antibiotics. Post-partum
investigation with an IVP is not necessary. It is associated with preterm labour but
does not cause neonatal death.

Reference
Davison J. Renal disease. In: De Swiet M, ed. *Medical Disorders in Obstetrics Practice*,
2nd edn. Oxford: Blackwell Scientific Publications, 1990; 306–407.

Eclampsia
182, 186   (Pre-eclampsia, eclampsia and phaeochromocytoma)

The incidence of eclampsia is 44% post-partum, 38% ante-partum and 18% intra-partum. Use of hydralazine with chlormethiazole is not contraindicated. ARDS is the commonest cause of death. Oliguria is a feature not diuresis. The blood volume is decreased. Time and mode of delivery depends on the clinical situation. IV hydralazine or labetalol are used to control the raised blood pressure at first instance.

Reference
Redman C. Hypertension in pregnancy. In: De Swiet M, ed. *Medical Disorders in Obstetrics Practice*, 2nd edn. Oxford: Blackwell Scientific Publications, 1990; 249–305.

GnRH agonists are used effectively in the treatment of
193, 195, 196, 197

They are also used in the treatment of leiomyomas, endometriosis, hirsutism, functional bowel disease, menstrual asthma and migraine, dysfunctional bleeding, PCO and prior to endometrial resection/ablation

Reference
Pickersgill A. GnRH analogues and add-back therapy. Is there a perfect combination? *British Journal of Obstetrics and Gynaecology*, 1998; **105**: 475–485.

Maternal CVS in pregnancy
201   (Cardiac disease in pregnancy)

Heart murmurs are due to increased blood flow through the internal mammary arteries. Anticoagulants should not be stopped at 36 weeks because of the high risk of thrombosis. Benzyl penicillin plus gentamycin provides adequate prophylaxis. Frusemide is essential in the management of heart failure, but it is not advocated in the initial management of eclampsia.

Reference
Whitfield CR. Heart disease in pregnancy. In: Whitfield CR, ed. *Dewhurst's Textbook of Obstetrics and Gynaecology for Postgraduates*, 5th edn. Oxford: Blackwell Science, 1995; 216–227.

The following are true when comparing modern obstetric practices regarding instrumental deliveries
203, 204, 205   (Forceps and ventouse)

For vaginal delivery neither instrument should be used (in modern obstetric practice) unless the cervix is fully dilated (forceps may be used in Caesarean section).

Vaginal pH
207, 210, 211

At birth neonatal vaginal pH is lowest due to the effect of maternal hormones and it gradually increases thereafter. Both cervical and menstrual discharges are alkaline and therefore increase vaginal pH. Oestrogen replacement therapy decreases vaginal pH.

References
Emens JM. Intractable vaginal discharge. *Current Obstetrics and Gynaecology*, 1993;
    3: 41–47.
Lamont RF. Bacterial vaginosis. *The Year Book of the RCOG 1994*; 149–158.
Whitfield, CR, ed. *Dewhurst's Textbook of Obstetrics and Gynaecology for*
    Postgraduates. 5th edn. Oxford: Blackwell Science, 1995; 4–53.

Predisposing factors to face presentation include
213, 214, 215, 216, 217, 218, 219, 220   (Presentations and positions)
Others are sternomastoid tumour, branchial cyst, contracted pelvis, pelvic tumour,
fetal goitre, large thorax, cord around the neck etc.

Reference
Ritchie JWK. Malpositions of the occiput and malpresentations. In: Whitfield CR, ed.
    Dewhurst's Textbook of Obstetrics and Gynaecology for Postgraduates, 5th edn. Oxford:
    Blackwell Science, 1995; 346–367.

The following are not associated with hirsutism
223   (Hirsutism)
Anorexia nervosa, hyperthecosis of the ovary, acromegaly, juvenile hypothyroidism
and hilar cell tumours are associated with hirsutism.

Reference
Davies MC, Jacobs HS. Hirsutism. RCOG PACE review 95/11.

Ovarian tumours may be associated with
227, 228, 229   (Ovarian tumours: non-epithelial)
There is no association with Kallman's syndrome.

Reference
Eccles DM. Ovarian cancer genetics and screening for ovarian cancer. RCOG PACE
    review 97/06.

Massive obstetric haemorrhage
233, 234
Initially blood loss should be replaced by blood. Platelets and fresh frozen plasma are
needed if coagulation failure develops.

Reference
Annexe to Chapter 3. *Report on Confidential Enquiries into Maternal Deaths in the*
    United Kingdom, 1988–1990. London: HMSO, 1994.

Progestogens, when given with oestrogens to post-menopausal women
238, 240
Increase LDL cholesterol, cause endometrial down-regulation, have no preventive effect on breast cancer (may increase the risk) and do not act as insulin antagonists. Although the mechanisms are unclear, progestogens do reduce bone loss.

Deep venous thrombosis (DVT) and pregnancy
242, 243   (Coagulation and pregnancy)
80% of DVTs occur in the left leg. This is associated with a 16% risk of pulmonary embolism, the risk being highest during first 24 hours after the primary thrombotic episode. Pulmonary embolism can occur as a primary event.

Reference
Report on Confidential Enquiries into Maternal Deaths in the United Kingdom, 1991–
    1993. London: HMSO, 1996.

Recognized features of Turner's syndrome include
247, 248, 249, 250
They are infertile, have raised gonadotrophins secondary to ovarian failure and can only conceive with donor eggs. The majority are XO (associated with chromatin negative buccal cells) although about 10% are associated with the mosaic pattern XO/XX. Anosmia is associated with Kallman's syndrome. Their bone age is delayed for their age. Red–green colour blindness is associated with the absence of one X chromosome.

The menstrual cycle
254, 258, 259, 260   (Infertility - I, Menstrual cycle physiology)
Even in normal cycles the average length of the luteal phase is 12–15 days. Ovulation occurs on average 32 hours after the initial LH rise and 16.5 hours after the LH peak. Although a day 21 progesterone is used to diagnose ovulation, it only implies adequate corpus luteal functioning and is therefore an indirect method. Unless follicular tracking occurs at the same time cases of luteinized unruptured follicle (LUF) will be missed. Thecal cells of the ovarian stroma mainly secrete androstenedione but can secrete oestrogens.

Intrauterine contraceptive devices (IUCD)
263, 264, 267, 270, 271   (Contraception and sterilization)
Levonorgestrel releasing IUCD (LNG-IUCD) do not contain copper and do not need removal prior to an MRI. They should be removed post-menopausally as there is a theoretical risk of pyometra. They are not advised for renal transplant patients who require immunosuppressive therapy because of the theoretical risks of ascending infection. Efficacy is unrelated to the weight of copper, but is proportional to the surface area of the copper. Protection from the ectopic pregnancy is less effective (95%).

In rupture of the uterus, the following may occur
272, 274, 275, 276
Other features are constant lower abdominal pain without any uterine contractions, maternal tachycardia, abnormal cardiotocography etc. The uterine contractions usually stop after rupture of the uterus.

Reference
Beazley JM. Maternal injuries and complications. In: Whitfield CR, ed. *Dewhurst's Textbook of Obstetrics and Gynaecology for Postgraduates*, 5th edn. Oxford: Blackwell Science, 1995; 377–387.

Causes of pruritus ani include
277, 279, 281
Ascaris is a roundworm – only threadworms (in the young) cause pruritus. Diverticulitis does not cause pruritus ani. Other causes are lack of cleanliness, excessive sweating, wearing rough or woollen underclothing, anal or perianal discharge, vaginal discharge (e.g. Trichomonas vaginalis), scabies, pediculosis, epidermophytosis, allergy, psoriasis, lichen planus, contact dermatitis, intertrigo, psychoneurosis etc.

Reference
The rectum. The anus and anal canal. In: Mann CV, Russell RCG, eds. *Bailey & Love's Short Practice of Surgery*, 21st edn. London: Chapman & Hall, 1992; 1215–1239, 1240–1275.

SLE in pregnancy
282, 283, 284   (Immunology of pregnancy)
There is a high risk of puerperal exacerbation as the immunosuppressive action of pregnancy is withdrawn. The disease causes microthrombosis of the placenta increasing the risk of spontaneous miscarriage and pre-eclampsia. Azathioprine may be used if required. Lupus anticoagulant increases the risk of thrombosis.

Reference
Jones WR. Immunological disorders in pregnancy. In: Whitfield CR, ed. *Dewhurst's Textbook of Obstetrics and Gynaecology for Postgraduates*, 5th edn. Oxford: Blackwell Science, 1995; 277–287.

The following conditions can be detected by ultrasound scanning
287, 288, 289, 290, 291
Duodenal atresia is seen as a double bubble sign. In hydrops fetalis, skin oedema and excessive collection of fluid in serous cavities are characteristic. Congenital heart block is diagnosed by the ventricles beating at a lower rate than the atria (atrio-ventricular dissociation).

Reference
Harman C. The routine 18–20 week ultrasound scan. In: James DK, Steer PJ, Weiner CP, Gonik B, eds. *High Risk Pregnancy Management Options*. London: WB Saunders Company, 1994; 661–691.

Regarding puberty
292, 294

Dural tap
295, 296, 297, 299
Post-dural puncture headache commonly occurs within 1–2 days. It is treated with a 'blood patch' which is effective immediately.

Reference
Collins RE, Morgan BM. Regional anaesthesia and obstetrics. *Current Obstetrics and Gynaecology*, 1995; **5**: 91–97.

PAPER TWO

Allow 2 hours for completion of this paper

Necrotizing enterocolitis in the newborn

1. Affects male infants more often than female
2. Is much more common among infants whose birth weight is less than 1500 g
3. The earliest sign is abdominal distension following initiation of oral feeding
4. *E. coli* is the commonest organism recovered from blood cultures
5. Thrombocytopenia is the rule
6. Bilious vomiting is found
7. Intestinal obstruction is a characteristic feature
8. Bloody diarrhoea occurs
9. Gas in the bowel wall on abdominal X-ray is diagnostic

A 24-year-old primigravida at 37 weeks gestation has had a blood pressure of 150/100 mm Hg and 4 g of proteinuria for the preceding day. The following findings would be expected

10. A raised plasma urate level
11. Loss of diurnal variation in blood pressure
12. A creatinine clearance of 120–150 ml per minute
13. Hyperreflexia
14. A low level of FDP
15. Hypernatraemia

The following are more common after an abdominal (rather than vaginal) hysterectomy

16. Lung atelectasis
17. Febrile morbidity
18. Pulmonary embolism

Monozygotic multiple pregnancy

19. Is monoamniotic in 25% of cases
20. Incidences are more common in Japan than in North America
21. Incidences are more common in pregnancies conceived on clomiphene
22. The incidence increases with increasing maternal age
23. Such pregnancies are familial
24. Is the usual mechanism of conception in triplet pregnancies
25. Is associated with higher incidence of fetal abnormalities than polyzygotic pregnancies
26. Communicating vessels in the placenta are usually demonstrated

Depo medroxyprogesterone acetate

27. Is the only available licensed depot contraceptive preparation
28. Is associated with significant loss of bone mineral density in long-term users
29. The duration of its contraceptive efficacy is dose related
30. Induces amenorrhoea in 45% in the first year of use
31. Has androgenic side effects
32. Is contraindicated in women who have previously had an ectopic pregnancy
33. Is associated with reduced incidence of PID
34. Is contraindicated in sickle cell disease
35. Is discontinued by a third of users because of menstrual irregularities

Regarding miscarriage, which of the following statements are true?

36. One in four women will have at least one miscarriage
37. One in five first trimester miscarriages are associated with chromosomal anomalies
38. One in 100 women experience recurrent miscarriage
39. One in five women experience vaginal bleeding in early pregnancy
40. One in three spontaneous miscarriages will resolve spontaneously

In pregnancy

41. The incidence of appendicitis is 1 in 2500
42. Pancreatitis is associated with 50% mortality
43. Asymptomatic bacteriuria may presents with suprapubic pain
44. Nephrolithiasis occurs in 1 in 5000–10 000 cases
45. Sickle cell disease may present with sharp abdominal pain

In labour

46. Uterine hypertonia is the commonest type of abnormal uterine activity
47. Uterine hypotonia is commoner in parous than in primigravidae
48. Supine position is associated with uterine hypotonia
49. Adequate pain relief may correct uterine hypertonia
50. Uterine hypotonia is associated with fetal hypoxia

The following indicate abnormal sperm function

51. Volume <2 ml
52. Density of 10 million/ml
53. 70% abnormal forms
54. Motility 40%

Short stature is associated with

55. Androgen insensitivity
56. Klippel–Feil syndrome
57. Turner's syndrome
58. XXX genotype

There is a recognized association between Down's syndrome and

59. Congenital deafness
60. Patent ductus arteriosus
61. 21 triploidy
62. Hypotonia
63. 13/21 translocation defect

The following side effects match

64. Digoxin   Agranulocytosis
65. Methyldopa   Depression
66. Warfarin   Osteoporosis
67. Clomiphene   Alopecia
68. Cimetidine   Mastalgia
69. Norethisterone   Neonatal virilism
70. Danazol   Acne
71. Bromocriptine   Hypertension

Regarding contraception in late reproductive life

72. At 50 years of age the pregnancy rate in women not using any contraception is 10–20 per 100 women years
73. Contraception should be discontinued with the last menstrual period if this has occurred after the age of 50
74. Contraception should be discontinued 1 year after the last menstrual period if this has occurred before the age of 50
75. Methods of contraception with a high failure rate in young women are more reliable in the peri-menopausal period
76. The indications and contraindications for post-coital contraception are exactly the same in peri-menopausal women as for younger age groups
77. Modern low dose combined oral contraceptive pills can be taken in healthy non-smoking women in the peri-menopausal age range
78. Modern cyclical and continuous combined hormone replacement therapy provides reliable contraception
79. Older women have the highest incidence of therapeutic abortion of any age group

New genetics

80. The majority of mutations causing genetic diseases are single base substitutions
81. There is a specific base substitution with genes in all genetic disorders
82. Restriction endonucleases always cut DNA strands at the same point
83. Restriction enzymes are useful in diagnosing sickle cell disease
84. Introns are important in coding for genetic products
85. All patients with alpha-1-antitrypsin deficiency have the same underlying base substitution

ARDS

86. Is rarely associated with sepsis
87. Is commonly associated with aspiration of gastric contents
88. Is associated with multiple blood transfusions in only 25% of cases
89. Develops within 24 hours in 80% of patients
90. Mortality rates vary according to the underlying cause

Presumptive evidence of ovulation is indicated by

91. A biphasic temperature chart during a menstrual cycle
92. The development of subnuclear vacuolation in the endometrial glands
93. A rise in urinary LH
94. A fall in urinary pregnanediol excretion during the third week
95. The development of supranuclear vacuolation in the endometrial glands

Listeria monocytogenes in pregnancy

96. Is destroyed by cooking
97. Causes a glandular fever-like illness
98. Severe diarrhoea is characteristic
99. Is best treated with chloramphenicol
100. Is a cause of recurrent miscarriage
101. May result in neonatal hydrocephalus
102. Causes meconium ileus

Pelvic abscess is a recognized complication of

103. Diverticulitis coli
104. Crohn's disease
105. Ulcerative colitis
106. Appendicitis
107. Schistosoma hematobium infestation
108. Pyometra

The following are associated with an increased risk of fetal malformations

109. Diagnostic amniocentesis
110. Poliomyelitis vaccine administered in early pregnancy

Characteristic features of primary spasmodic dysmenorrhoea include

111. Relief of pain by mefenamic acid
112. Endometrium in the secretory phase
113. Mildly elevated serum prolactin levels
114. Ovulation
115. Excess production of $PGF_{2\alpha}$ by the endometrium
116. Increased production of parathormone

Genetic counselling includes

117. An attempt to eliminate hereditary disease
118. Always offering chorionic villus sampling (CVS)

Which of the following associations are correct

119.	46 XXX	Super female
120.	47 XXY	Testicular feminization syndrome
121.	46 XX	True hermaphroditism
122.	46 XY/47 XXY	Klinefelter's syndrome
123.	47 XXX	Tall stature
124.	46 XO	Turner's syndrome
125.	46 XX	Female adrenogenital syndrome

Ectopic pregnancy

126. The incidence has been declining in the UK over the last few years
127. In the UK the incidence is 1/500 births
128. Following one ectopic pregnancy the risk of a further ectopic pregnancy is 40–50%
129. The incidence of maternal deaths due to ectopic pregnancy in the UK in 1991–93 was 0.3/1000

Regarding drugs in the neonate, the following match

130. Phenytoin   Jaundice
131. Rifampicin   Hypoprothrombinaemia
132. Tetracycline   Discolouration, dysplasia of teeth and bones
133. Lithium   Retention of urine
134. Maloprim   Steven Johnson syndrome
135. Streptomycin   Deafness due to VIIth nerve damage
136. Tctracyclinc   Cataract

Peripartum cardiomyopathy

137. Persisting cardiomegaly at 1 year is associated with mortality of over 80%
138. Most commonly occurs post-partum
139. Is more common with multiple pregnancies, eclampsia and nulliparity
140. Normally presents with signs of right sided heart failure
141. May necessitate heart transplantation
142. Heparin is advised to reduce emboli

Causes of raised HCG include

143. Carcinoma of the colon
144. All forms of trophoblastic disease
145. Carcinoma of the bronchus
146. Carcinoma of the bladder
147. Carcinoma of the stomach

CIN 3 is characterized by

148. Visible lesions at colposcopy
149. Histological changes beneath the basement membrane
150. Full thickness loss of stratification throughout the epithelium
151. Full thickness loss of polarity throughout the epithelium
152. Lymph node deposits

Oligohydramnios is characteristically associated with

153. Post-maturity
154. Amniotic bands
155. Fetal polycystic kidneys
156. Rhesus alloimmunization
157. Haemangioma of the placenta
158. Diabetes mellitus
159. Increased levels of amniotic prolactin
160. A reduced efficiency of labour
161. All cases of renal agenesis of the fetus

The levonorgestrel loaded IUCD

162. Effectively improves dysmenorrhoea
163. Does not alter the serum lipid profile
164. May reduce the size of fibroids
165. Retains contraceptive efficacy for up to 3 years
166. Is associated with significant weight gain
167. Reduces menstrual blood loss by up to 95% after 1 year of use

In amniotic fluid

168. Presence of phosphatidyl inositol indicates fetal lung maturity
169. A lecithin–sphingomyelin ratio of 2:1 indicates fetal lung maturity in maternal diabetes
170. Absence of phosphatidyl glycerol indicates that the fetal lung is immature
171. Phospholipids make up more than 80% of surfactant
172. Lecithin contributes about 80% of surfactant after 37 weeks gestation

The following fall after the menopause

173. Serum testosterone levels
174. Plasma calcium concentration
175. Karyopyknotic index in the vagina
176. HDL and coronary heart disease
177. Plasma oestradiol concentrations
178. Urinary calcium/creatinine ratio
179. Interest in sexual intercourse

In pregnancy above 35 years old the incidence of the following are increased

180. Post-maturity
181. Anencephaly
182. Breech presentation
183. Perinatal death
184. Closed spina bifida
185. Monozygotic twins
186. IUGR
187. Prolonged labour

Toxoplasmosis infection in pregnancy

188. Occurs from improperly washed raw vegetables
189. Can be effectively treated in pregnancy
190. The fetus is affected in less than 5% cases
191. Less than 20% of fetuses are affected if the mother was affected in previous pregnancies
192. 80% of fetuses are affected if infection occurs in the first or second trimester
193. Causes abortion in 20–30% of cases
194. Causes jaundice on the first day of life

The following statements relate to pelvic inflammatory disease (PID)

195. 8% of women suffer with tubal factor infertility after one episode
196. 40% of women suffer with tubal factor infertility after three or more episodes
197. 1% of women are infertile after one episode of mild disease
198. 20% are infertile after the first episode of severe disease
199. 1% with laparoscopically proven PID have Fitz–Hugh–Curtis syndrome
200. 3% will have another episode within a year
201. 80% of partners of women with PID will have urethritis

Folic acid deficiency in pregnancy

202. Is more likely to occur in women of low social class
203. Is associated with Hirshsprung's disease
204. Has no known association with Crohn's disease
205. Causes fetal neural tube defects

With regard to ovarian carcinoma the following screening methods are beneficial

206. Ultrasound using colour flow doppler
207. CA 125
208. Genetics

Pethidine

209. The maximum dose is 400 mg in 24 hours, and it should be entirely avoided in pre-eclampsia
210. Delayed gastric emptying, nausea, vomiting and maternal respiratory depression are known side effects
211. If given in labour, prophylactic ranitidine should be administered concurrently

The following drugs are associated with hirsutism

212. Phenytoin
213. Diazoxide
214. Salicylate
215. Digoxin
216. Cimetidine

Placenta praevia

217. Occurs in 2–4% of pregnancies
218. Occurs with higher incidence in women who have previously had a D&C
219. Is associated with an increased incidence of neonatal respiratory distress syndrome
220. Classically presents with painless antepartum haemorrhage late in the second trimester
221. One in three women with placenta praevia have no history of antepartum haemorrhage
222. Always necessitates Caesarean delivery
223. Is associated with maternal mortality of 0.1%
224. Is associated with placenta acreta in 15%

Atelectasis

225. Is a rare postoperative complication after general anaesthesia
226. Has a more aggressive course in non-smokers than smokers
227. May present with pyrexia
228. The risk increases with increased duration of anaesthesia

Breech delivery

229. Footling breech presentation is an indication for Caesarean section
230. Vaginal delivery is impossible if the maternal sacrum is flat
231. Ideally the membranes should be kept intact during labour for as long as possible
232. In primigravida a trial of labour is contraindicated
233. The risk of cord prolapse in labour is highest in flexed breech
234. Breech extraction in singleton pregnancy is contraindicated
235. The after-coming head entrapped with an incompletely dilated cervix could be released with incisions at 6 and 12 o'clock
236. In the early 1990s Caesarean sections for breeches in England accounted for 30% of all Caesarean sections
237. Pushing should commence as soon as full dilatation is achieved

A 32-year-old woman, para 4 + 0 has requested a sterilization. She is rather overweight and is found to have second degree uterine prolapse. Routine cervical cytology has shown severe dyskaryosis, confirmed as CIN 3 by colposcopic biopsy. Acceptable management for this woman could be

238. Sterilization and treatment of the cervix
239. Abdominal hysterectomy
240. Manchester repair with sterilization
241. Schauta's operation
242. Cone biopsy

Transverse lie in late pregnancy is associated with

243. Renal agenesis
244. IUGR
245. Microcephaly
246. Placenta circumvallata
247. Haemangioma of the placenta
248. Arcuate uterus
249. Multiple pregnancy
250. Placenta praevia

Precocious puberty

251. Can be treated with cyproterone acetate
252. Is rarely of the familial constitutional type
253. Is associated with Albright's syndrome
254. Is associated with juvenile hypothyroidism
255. Is associated with granulosa cell tumours
256. Is associated with sarcoma botryoides
257. Is associated with Waterhouse–Friedrichsen's syndrome

Recognized causes of post-partum shock without excessive visible blood loss include

258. Inversion of the uterus
259. Intravenous administration of ergometrine
260. Rupture of the uterus
261. Vaginal haematoma
262. An eclamptic fit

Partial moles

263. Incidence in the UK is 1 in 600 deliveries
264. 5% of patients will need treatment for persistent trophoblastic disease
265. Do not need follow up with serial HCG
266. May be associated with fetal erythrocytes
267. Are triploid (one paternal, two maternal)

Ovarian hyperstimulation syndrome may be associated with

268. Clomiphene tartrate
269. Human menopausal gonadotrophins
270. FSH
271. Tamoxifen
272. HCG

Right iliac fossa (RIF) pain occurring at 32 weeks of pregnancy could be due to

273. Constipation
274. Chronic salpingitis
275. A strangulated femoral hernia

Heparin

276. When used in prophylactic doses does not require monitoring of clotting
277. For therapeutic use, its anticoagulant effect is monitored by measuring PT
278. The target level of PT for a woman on a therapeutic dose of heparin is 1.5–2 times normal
279. Osteopenia due to prolonged heparin therapy is reversible after discontinuation of the treatment
280. The disadvantage of the low molecular weight heparin is a higher incidence of allergic reactions when compared with unfractionated heparin
281. The APTT should be measured 12 hours after starting intravenous heparin therapy
282. Heparin associated thrombocytopenia could be life threatening
283. Epidural anaesthesia is safe in women on prophylactic dose of unfractionated heparin

The transformation zone of the cervix

284. Is entirely visible when colposcopy is regarded adequate
285. Is the usual site for the development of CIN
286. Has the squamo-columnar junction at its ectocervical limit
287. May extend to include the vagina in 5% of patients
288. Only contains columnar cells
289. May contain dysplastic cells

Breast cancer in pregnancy

290. Is characterized by a worse prognosis if it occurs during or shortly after pregnancy
291. Could be treated with radiotherapy
292. In pregnancy there is a preponderance of unfavourable types of breast cancer
293. Pregnancy after breast cancer should be delayed for 2 years because of the poor prognosis
294. Breast feeding is not advisable

Urinary retention

295. Is a common gynaecological problem
296. Is a side effect of cholinergic drugs
297. Is a common complication of early pregnancy
298. Could be caused by primary syphilis
299. Could be caused by genital herpes
300. Could be caused by regional anaesthesia

ANSWERS TO PAPER TWO

The numbers of the correct answers are given

Necrotizing enterocolitis in the newborn
1, 2, 3, 4, 5, 6, 8, 9
Intestinal obstruction is not a feature.

References
Cockburn F. Neonatal care for obstetricians. In: Whitfield CR, ed. *Dewhurst's Textbook of Obstetrics and Gynaecology for Postgraduates*, 5th edn. Oxford: Blackwell Science, 1995; 454–476.
Necrotising enterocolitis. In: Chamberlain GVP, ed. *Obstetrics by Ten Teachers*, 16th edn. London: Edward Arnold, 1995; 318.

In proteinuric hypertension the following findings would be expected
10, 11, 13 15   (Pre-eclampsia, eclampsia and phaeochromocytoma)
The creatinine clearance would be expected to be low (normal: 90–120 ml/min) and the FDP level would be higher.

Reference
Redman C. Hypertension in pregnancy. In: De Swiet M, ed. *Medical Disorders in Obstetrics Practice*, 2nd edn. Oxford: Blackwell Scientific Publications, 1990; 249–305.

The following are more common after an abdominal (rather than vaginal) hysterectomy
16, 17, 18   (Abdominal versus vaginal hysterectomy)
Unintended visceral damage occurs more often with vaginal surgery.

Monozygotic multiple pregnancy
25, 26   (Multiple pregnancy)
Only 3% of monozygotic twins are monoamniotic. The incidence is not influenced by geographical area, ovulation induction, maternal age, family etc. (which do influence polyzygotic pregnancies). Triplets are usually polyzygotic.

Reference
Neilson JP. Multiple pregnancy. In: Whitfield CR, ed. *Dewhurst's Textbook of Obstetrics and Gynaecology for Postgraduates*, 5th edn. Oxford: Blackwell Science, 1995; 439–453.

Depo medroxyprogesterone acetate
29, 30, 31, 33, 35   (Contraception and sterilization)
Norethisterone oenanthate is an alternative. Depo-provera reduces the incidence of
the sickle cell crisis, and is not associated with significant bone mineral loss.

References
Globade B, Ellis S, Murby B, Randall S, Kirkman R. Bone density in long term users
    of depot medroxyprogesterone acetate. *British Journal of Obstetrics and
    Gynaecology*, 1998; **105**: 790–794.
Walling M. Injectable and implant contraceptives. In: *Contraception*. (Update
    Postgraduate Centre Series), Reed Healthcare Communications, 1995; 22–24.

Regarding miscarriage, which of the following statements are true?
36, 38, 39   (Abortion spontaneous/recurrent)
Up to 50% of first trimester miscarriages are associated with chromosomal
abnormalities. 70% of spontaneous miscarriages will resolve spontaneously.

In pregnancy
41, 45   (Abdominal pain in pregnancy)
The mortality associated with pancreatitis is 10%. As the name of the condition
indicates, asymptomatic bacteriuria is asymptomatic. If symptoms such as suprapubic
pain intervene urinary tract infection needs to be considered. The incidence of
nephrolithiasis is 1:1500.

Reference
Stabile I, Chard T, Grudzinskas G. *Clinical Obstetrics and Gynaecology*. New York:
    Springer-Verlag, 1996; 113–114.

In labour
48, 49   (Abnormal uterine function in labour)
Hypotonia is the commonest type of abnormal uterine activity. It is commoner in
primigravid women although can occur in parous ones. It is not known to be
associated with fetal hypoxia.

Reference
Arulkumaran S. Poor progress in labour including augmentation, malpositions and
    malpresentations. In: James DK, Steer PJ, Weiner CP, Gonik B. eds. *High Risk
    Pregnancy. Management Options*. London: WB Saunders Company, 1994; 1061–1075.

The following indicate abnormal sperm function
(Male subfertility)
The values are all abnormal for semen analysis, but it is argued that semen analysis
does not test sperm function—some men with normal semen analysis are infertile.
Sperm function can be tested by the capacitation test or the hamster oocyte
penetration test. (Normal semen analysis values are: volume 2–5 ml, density 20–100
million/ml, <50% abnormal forms and motility >50%.)

Short stature is associated with
57
Androgen insensitivity and XXX genotype result in tall females. Klippel–Feil syndrome is associated with a short, webbed neck but not stature.

There is a recognized association between Down's syndrome and
62   (Prenatal diagnosis)
Down's syndrome is a chromosomal disorder caused by trisomy 21 due to non-disjunction (95–98%) and 14/21, 21/22 and 21/21 translocations (2–5%). This syndrome is associated with mental retardation, brachycephaly, microcephaly, mongoloid facies, endocardial cushion defects (e.g. ASD), duodenal atresia (double bubble sign at scan), single palmer crease, short middle phalanx of the fifth finger, infertile boys, subfertile girls etc. Cardiac defects (present in 40%) are the main cause of early death.

References
James D. Genetic counselling. In: James DK, Steer PJ, Weiner CP, Gonik B, eds. *High Risk Pregnancy Management Options*. London: WB Saunders Company,1994; 9-20.
Neilson JP. Antenatal diagnosis of fetal abnormality. In: Whitfield CR, ed. *Dewhurst's Textbook of Obstetrics and Gynaecology for Postgraduates*, 5th edn. Oxford: Blackwell Science, 1995; 121–139.

The following side effects match
65, 67, 69, 70
Digoxin may cause gastro-intestinal side effects and cardiac arrythmias but it is not associated with agranulocytosis. Heparin (not warfarin) is a cause of osteoporosis. Cimetidine does not cause mastalgia, but may cause gynaecomastia, agranulocytosis and impotence. Danazol causes acne in the user and may cause virilism of a female fetus. Bromocriptine causes hypotension.

Reference
British National Formulary, **35**; March 1998.

Regarding contraception in late reproductive life
75, 76, 77
The pregnancy rate is 0–5 pregnancies per 100 women years. Contraception should be continued for 1 year after the last menstrual period in the over 50 age group. It should be continued for 2 years after the last menstrual period in this under 50 age group. HRT has no contraceptive action.

References
Cogswell D, Randall S. Contraceptive advice for the perimenopausal woman. *Trends in Urology, Gynaecology and Sexual Health*. November/December, 1996; 46–54.
Gebbie A. Contraception for the over forties. *Progress* **12**: 293–308.
Harper C. Contraception in the perimenopause. In: *Contraception* (Update Postgraduate Centre Series), Reed Healthcare Communications, 1995; 54–57.

Genetics

80, 83

The nucleotide bases of DNA are adenine, guanine, cytosine and thymidine. Bands in DNA occur between adenine and guanine, and cytosine and thymidine. Although the majority of genetic mutations are single base substitutions, more subtle rearrangements of a gene may alter the structure of the mRNA and the protein synthesis. Restriction endonucleases cut DNA at different sites. Exons are important in coding for genetic products. Alpha-1-antitrypsin is the product of a highly polymorphic gene locus called PI (protease inhibitor) containing about 75 alleles. The common or wild-type form of alpha-antitrypsin is called PI-M.

Reference

Weatherall DJ. *The New Genetics and Clinical Practice*, 3rd edn. Oxford: Oxford University Press, 1991; 39–102, 138–192.

ARDS

87, 88, 89, 90 (Perioperative complications in obstetrics and gynaecology, Report on Confidential Enquiries into Maternal Deaths in the United Kingdom 1991–1993) ARDS is commonly associated with sepsis (30–40% of cases) and aspiration of gastric contents (30–35% of cases). Mortality rates vary e.g. high (90%) with sepsis, low (10%) with fat embolism.

Presumptive evidence of ovulation is indicated by

91, 92, 93, 95 (Menstrual cycle physiology)

Urinary pregnanediol excretion during the third week would be expected to rise.

Listeria monocytogenes in pregnancy

96, 97, 101, 102 (Infection in pregnancy)

Listeria is associated with inadequately heated/reheated and cold foods. During pregnancy it most commonly affects the mother in the third trimester and may initially present as a flu-like illness (fever, backache, myalgia), if the backache is prominent it may mimic a UTI. It is occasionally associated with gastro-intestinal disturbances. Ampicillin is the drug of choice. It may cause an occasional miscarriage, but it is not a cause of recurrent miscarriages. In the affected neonate it may cause jaundice, purulent conjunctivitis, broncho-pneumonia, meningitis and encephalitis. It is associated with meconium-stained liquor.

Reference

The Chief Medical Officer. The diagnosis and treatment of suspected listeriosis in pregnancy. *Report of a Working Group, 1992*. PL/CMO (92) 19.

Pelvic abscess is a recognized complication of

103, 104, 105, 106, 107 (Pelvic inflammatory disease)

Pyometra is usually an infection confined to the uterine cavity.

The following are associated with an increased risk of fetal malformations
109 (Prenatal diagnosis)
Amniocentesis is associated with orthopaedic deformities. Other associations include paternal age over 50 (autosomal dominant mutations), advanced maternal age (chromosomal defects), maternal chronic alcoholism and a single umbilical artery (single umbilical vein is not). Poliomyelitis vaccine is not associated with fetal malformations.

References
MacLean AB and Cockburn F. Maternal and perinatal infection. In: Whitfield CR, ed. *Dewhurst's Textbook of Obstetrics and Gynaecology for Postgraduates*, 5th edn. Oxford: Blackwell Science, 1995; 477–493.
Wilkins-Haug L. Genetic disease and the fetus. In: Frederickson HL, Wilkins-Haug L, eds. *Ob/Gyn Secrets*. Philadelphia: Hanley & Belfus, Inc., 1991; 207–210.

Characteristic features of primary spasmodic dysmenorrhoea include
111, 112, 114, 115
It is associated with the ovulatory cycle and increased production of $PGF_{2\alpha}$ in the endometrium. There is no association with prolactin or parathormone.

Genetic counselling includes
Taking a detailed family history, discussing prenatal diagnosis, interpreting karyotypic reports etc. It neither attempts to eliminate hereditary disease through counselling nor always offer CVS or amniocentesis.

Reference
James D. Genetic counselling. In: James DK, Steer PJ, Weiner CP, Gonik B, eds. *High Risk Pregnancy Management Options*. London: WB Saunders Company, 1994; 9–20.

Which of the following associations are correct
121, 122, 123, 125
47XXX is a super female. Testicular feminization is 46 XY. Turner's syndrome is 45 XO.

Reference
Neilson JP. Antenatal diagnosis of fetal abnormality. In: Whitfield CR, ed. *Dewhurst's Textbook of Obstetrics and Gynaecology for Postgraduates*, 5th edn, Oxford: Blackwell Science, 1995; 221–239.

Ectopic pregnancy
129 (Ectopic pregnancy)
Although declining incidence is true of Scandinavia the incidence in the UK has been increasing. The incidence is 1:150 births. The risk of a further ectopic pregnancy is 15%.

Drugs in the neonate – match
130, 131, 132, 133, 134, 136 (Drugs in pregnancy)
Streptomycin can cause deafness due to VIIIth nerve damage.

Peripartum cardiomyopathy
138, 141, 142
This rare condition (1/1 300–4000 deliveries) has a peak incidence 1–2 months post-partum. If cardiomegaly persists at 5 years mortality is in excess of 80%. It is more common with multiple pregnancies, eclampsia and multiparity in women over 30 years. It normally presents with signs of congestive cardiac failure (fatigue, breathlessness and oedema). It can be associated with emboli so some advise heparin prophylaxis. Treatment is supportive with anti-hypertensives and diuretics. If treatment fails heart transplantation may be necessary.

Reference
Morrison WL, Petch MC. Peripartum cardiomyopathy. *Hospital update.* 1991. 693–698.

Causes of raised HCG include
143, 144, 145, 146, 147

CIN 3 is characterized by
148, 150, 151   (Premalignant disease of the cervix)
Lymph node deposits and invasion through the basement membrane imply carcinoma. There are no histological changes beneath the basement membrane.

Oligohydramnios is characteristically associated with
153, 154, 155   (Polyhydramnios/oligohydramnios)
Oligohydramnios is also associated with IUGR (83%), increased fetal distress in labour and meconium aspiration.

Reference
Stark C. Disorders of the amniotic fluid. In: Frederickson HL, Wilkins-Haug L, eds. *Ob/Gyn Secrets.* Philadelphia: Hanley & Belfus, Inc., 1991; 217–220.

The levonorgestrel loaded IUCD
162, 163, 164, 167   (Contraception and sterilization)
Retains contraceptive efficacy for 5–8 years. There is no evidence to support weight gain.

References
Luukkainen T. The levonorgestrel-releasing IUD. *The British Journal of Family Planning,* 1993; **19**: 221–224.
Sturridge F, Guillebaud J. Gynaecological aspects of levonorgestrel-releasing intrauterine system. *British Journal of Obstetrics and Gynaecology,* 1997; **104**: 285–289.

In amniotic fluid
170, 171, 172
Phosphatidyl glycerol indicates lung maturity. A lecithin-sphingomyelin ratio of 2:1 indicates fetal lung maturity and this is usually reached by 33–34 weeks. Despite an adequate ratio, maturation delay is found in maternal diabetes, renal disease and identical twins.

References

Gibson AT. Surfactant and the neonatal lung. *British Journal of Hospital Medicine* 1997, **58**: 381–397.

Ritchie JWK. The fetus, placenta and amniotic fluid. In: Whitfield CR, ed. *Dewhurst's Textbook of Obstetrics and Gynaecology for Postgraduates*, 5th edn. Oxford: Blackwell Science, 1995; 73–86.

Roberton NRC. Developments in neonatal paediatric practice. In: Hull D, ed. *Recent Advances in Paediatrics, No. 6*. Edinburgh: Churchill Livingstone, 1981; 13-50.

The following fall after the menopause
175, 177, 179   (Menopause)
HDL falls but coronary heart disease increases. Urinary calcium/creatinine ratio increases in association with increasing bone metabolism. Free (serum) testosterone increases because of a fall in the levels of SHBG, but total testosterone levels are lower because of a decreased peripheral conversion of androstenedione.

In pregnancy above 35 years old the incidence of the following are increased
183, 187
There is no association with post-maturity, anencephaly, spina bifida, prolonged labour or breech. It is associated with dizygotic twins. Perinatal death is increased by three times. Other problems include increased hypertension and other medical problems, arthritis, thromboembolism, fibroids, chromosomal abnormality in the fetus, operative delivery (Caesarean section five times increase), preterm delivery (four times increase) etc.

Reference

Beazley JM. Special circumstances affecting labour. In: Whitfield CR, ed. *Dewhurst's Textbook of Obstetrics and Gynaecology for Postgraduates*, 5th edn. Oxford: Blackwell Science, 1995; 312–332.

Toxoplasmosis infection in pregnancy
188, 189, 191, 194   (Infection in pregnancy)
Toxoplasmosis is usually caused by ingestion of raw or undercooked meat, but it can occur from food contaminated by cat faeces. Effective treatment can be offered (drugs/termination). The chances of the fetus being affected are 6–15% in the first and 45–65% in the second trimester. Infection only occurs during the primary parasitaemia, so there is no risk from women who are seropositive or who have given birth to an affected baby previously. It rarely causes abortion.

References

Gravett MG, Sampson JE. Other infectious conditions. In: James DK, Steer PJ, Weiner CP, Gonik B, eds. *High Risk Pregnancy Management Options*. London: WB Saunders Company, 1994; 509–550.

MacLean AB, Cockburn F. Maternal and perinatal infection. In: Whitfield CR, ed. *Dewhurst's Textbook of Obstetrics and Gynaecology for Postgraduates*, 5th edn. Oxford: Blackwell Science, 1995; 477-493.

The following statements relate to pelvic inflammatory disease (PID)
195, 196, 197, 198, 201   (Pelvic inflammatory disease)
15% with laparoscopically proven PID have Fitz-Hugh–Curtis syndrome and 33% will have another episode within a year.

Reference
Bevan C. Pelvic inflammatory disease. RCOG PACE review 98/04.

Folic acid deficiency in pregnancy
202
Folate deficiency in pregnancy is known to be associated with anticonvulsant therapy, sickle cell disease, maternal megaloblastic anaemia, Crohn's disease, coeliac disease (not Hirshsprung's) and fetal abnormalities. Neural tube defects are associated with, not caused by, folate deficiency.

Reference
Letsky EA, Warwick R. Haematological problems. In: James DK, Steer PJ, Weiner CP, Gonik B. eds. *High Risk pregnancy Management Options*. London: WB Saunders Company, 1994; 337–372.

With regard to ovarian carcinoma the following screening methods are beneficial
Ultrasound using colour flow doppler is not specific. CA 125 is non-specific, but if elevated may act as a marker for recurrence. Only 5% of ovarian carcinomas are thought to arise by inheritance.

Pethidine
209, 210, 211   (Analgesia/anaesthesia in labour)
Pethidine is sedative. It is metabolized to norpethidine, which has convulsant properties so should be avoided in pre-eclampsia. Ranitidine or other antacids should be administered together with pethidine, because pethidine delays gastric emptying thus increasing the risk of Mendelson's syndrome.

References
British National Formulary **35**; March 1998
Morgan B. Maternal anaesthesia and analgesia in labour. In: James DK, Steer PJ, Weiner CP, Gonik B. eds. *High Risk Pregnancy Management Options*. London: WB Saunders Company, 1994; 1101–1118.

The following drugs are associated with hirsutism
212, 213, 215   (Hirsutism)

Placenta praevia
218, 219, 221, 223, 224   (Antepartum haemorrhage)
Placenta praevia occurs in less than 1% of pregnancies. Known associations include multiparity, previous Caesarean section and D&C. It classically presents with painless vaginal bleeding at 35 weeks. Maternal morbidity and mortality are increased. Fetal and neonatal complications include prematurity, IUGR, fetal anaemia, RDS (increased by 22%) and unexpected intrauterine death. Low grade placenta praevia is not a contraindication to vaginal delivery.

Reference
Stirrat GM. *Aids to Obstetrics and Gynaecology for MRCOG*, 4th edn. Churchill
    Livingstone, 1997; 118–120.

Atelectasis
227, 228   (Perioperative complications)
Atelectasis is common, especially in smokers where it is more aggressive. It may be associated with secondary infection.

Breech delivery
229, 231, 234   (Breech)
The risk of cord prolapse in labour is highest with footling breech presentation, hence the indication for caesarean section. Vaginal delivery in breech presentation is not impossible in women with a flat sacrum, but caution should be exercised as the risk of feto-pelvic disproportion is higher. Estimated fetal weight and pelvic dimensions are more important than primigravidity in predicting the chance of successful vaginal breech delivery. In labour the membranes should be kept intact for as long as possible. Pushing should also be delayed for as long as possible in order to avoid fetal head entrapment by an incompletely dilated cervix. If this occurs incisions at 4 and 8 o'clock should be made. In the early 90s Caesarean section in England for breech presentation accounted for 15% of all Caesareans.

Reference
Saunders NJ. The management of breech presentation. *British Journal of Hospital
    Medicine*, 1996; **56**(9): 456–458.

Acceptable management options following sterilization request by a 32-year-old woman with uterine prolapse and CIN 3
240
Sterilization and treatment of the cervix will not help with her prolapse, nor will a cone biopsy. Abdominal hysterectomy is less preferable than a vaginal hysterectomy and repair, and is associated with higher morbidity especially in overweight women. A radical hysterectomy of any sort (Wertheim's/Schauta's) is not indicated. It could be argued that vaginal hysterectomy is the only acceptable management option.

Transverse lie in late pregnancy is associated with

247, 248, 249, 250

Renal agenesis is associated with oligohydramnios. Others are prematurity (not IUGR), IUD, polyhydramnios, fundal attachment of the placenta, contracted pelvis, pelvic tumour, etc.

Reference

Ritchie JWK. Malpositions of the occiput and malpresentations. In: Whitfield CR, ed. *Dewhurst's Textbook of Obstetrics and Gynaecology for Postgraduates*, 5th edn. Oxford: Blackwell Science, 1995; 346–367.

Precocious puberty

251, 253, 255

The familial constitutional type accounts for the majority. It is associated with Albright's syndrome, does not lead to precocious sexual activity and can also be treated with GnRH analogues. Sarcoma botryoides, although found in children, is not a cause. Waterhouse–Friedrichsen's syndrome is associated with meningococcaemia. Hypothyroidism is associated with delayed puberty.

Recognized causes of post-partum shock without excessive visible blood loss include

258, 259, 260, 261, 262

Others are intravenous administration of local anaesthetics, myocardial infarction, diabetic coma, septic shock etc.

Reference

Duff P, Kopelman JN. Sudden postpartum collapse. In: Studd J, ed. *Progress in Obstetrics and Gynaecology*, Volume 6. Edinburgh: Churchill Livingstone, 1987; 223–240.

Partial moles

263, 266   (Gestational trophoblastic disease)

Partial moles are triploid (two paternal, one maternal). 0.5% will need treatment for persistent trophoblastic disease. They all need follow up with serial HCG.

Reference

Newlands ES. Trophoblastic disease. RCOG PACE review 96/10.

Ovarian hyperstimulation syndrome may be associated with

269, 270, 271, 272   (Infertility - II)

May also be associated with clomiphene citrate.

Reference

Management and prevention of ovarian hyperstimulation syndrome (OHSS). RCOG Guideline, 5 January 1995.

RIF pain occurring at 32 weeks of pregnancy could be due to
273, 275
Salpingitis does not occur during pregnancy. Femoral or inguinal hernias can present with pain.

Heparin
276, 279, 282, 283   (Coagulation and pregnancy)
Only therapeutic doses of heparin require monitoring. APTT is used to assess the therapeutic effect of heparin. APTT should be measured 4–6 hours after starting heparin therapy aiming for APTT ratio 1.5–2. Late onset (i.e. immunomediated) thrombocytopenia is associated with paradoxical thrombosis and could be life threatening. Low molecular weight heparin does not cause allergic reactions but may prolong the clotting time for longer and make epidurals relatively contraindicated.

References
Farquharson RG. Heparin, osteoporosis and pregnancy. *British Journal of Hospital Medicine*, 1997; **58**: 205–207.
Horn EH. Anticoagulants in pregnancy. *Current Obstetrics and Gynaecology*, 1996; **6**: 111–118.

The transformation zone of the cervix
284, 285, 287, 289   (Premalignant disease of the cervix)
The squamo-columnar junction is at its endocervical limit. It also contains squamous epithelium. Dysplasia is a histological diagnosis.

Breast cancer in pregnancy
290, 291, 292, 293   (Cancer in pregnancy)
Breast cancer in pregnancy is associated with early spread due to the increased blood supply, which adversely affects the prognosis. Radiotherapy is acceptable provided the fetus is adequately shielded. Pregnancy after breast cancer is allowed after 2 years (in the absence of recurrence) and has a good prognosis. There are no contraindications to breast feeding.

Reference
Pregnancy after breast cancer. RCOG Guideline 12, July 1997.

Urine retention
298, 299, 300   (Urinary incontinence: urodynamics)
This is a relatively rare problem in gynaecological practice. Besides the causes mentioned it can occur as a result of using anti-cholinergic drugs and pelvic masses obstructing the urethra.

Reference
Khullar V, Cardozo L. Drugs and bladder. *Current Obstetrics and Gynaecology*, 1995; **5**: 110–116.

PAPER THREE

Allow 2 hours for completion of this paper

Sickle cell disease in pregnancy

1. Is characterized by reduced globin molecule formation
2. In the UK, crisis occurs in 20% of pregnancies in affected women
3. In the UK, crisis is associated with 1–2% maternal mortality
4. Known complications include miscarriage, late fetal loss and type1 IUGR
5. Is associated with an increased incidence of urinary tract infection
6. The risk of sickle cell crisis could be reduced by using TED stockings, keeping the woman warm and well hydrated
7. Is a recognized contraindication to the use of prophylactic heparin in pregnancy
8. Spinal is preferred to epidural anaesthesia
9. Perinatal mortality rate in UK is 4–6 times greater than that of the normal population
10. Haemoglobin electrophoresis of the male partner of a woman with sickle cell trait is important before counselling
11. Antenatal diagnosis of sickle cell disease is currently available
12. The preferred mode of contraception for women with sickle cell disease is the IUCD

Colposcopy

13. Is only considered to be adequate if the upper margin of the transformation zone is completely seen
14. Glycogen is readily stained by iodine
15. Acetic acid causes protein coagulation in cells and thus white staining of the abnormal squamous epithelium
16. Colposcopically, HPV infection always shows features of intra-epithelial neoplasia
17. 'Schiller test negative' is synonymous with an iodine negative area
18. With increasing severity of intra-epithelial neoplasia, the punctuation becomes increasingly fine
19. Aceto-white changes indicate immature squamous metaplasia
20. Is an effective method in the diagnosis of VIN

Match the following oral contraceptive pills with their correct constituents

21. Marvelon	30 μg ethinyloestradiol	150 μg desogestrel
22. Microgynon	30 μg ethinyloestradiol	150 μg levonorgestrel
23. Neogest	30 μg ethinyloestradiol	250 μg levonorgestrel
24. Femodene	30 μg ethinyloestradiol	150 μg gestodene

Primary pruritus vulvae

25. Is commonly associated with perineal and anal itch
26. Is commonly caused by vaginal discharge
27. Improves at night
28. Vulval skin biopsy is mandatory for diagnosis
29. Psychological sequel are possible
30. Is commoner in young women

The Confidential Enquiries into Maternal Deaths in the United Kingdom (1991–93) reported that

31. The mortality rate following Caesarean section was 1/1000 operations
32. Avoidable factors were present in over 75% of anaesthetic deaths
33. The use of antacids regularly during labour protects against Mendelson's syndrome
34. More women died from post-partum haemorrhage than antepartum haemorrhage
35. 50% of deaths from amniotic fluid embolism occurred before the onset of labour

The risk of an endometrial cancer

36. In nulliparous women is twice that of a women with one child
37. Is raised in women on tamoxifen
38. Is increased in women with an early menarche
39. Is increased in women with a late menopause
40. Is decreased in women with diabetes mellitus
41. Is reduced by cigarette smoking
42. Is reduced by repeat prolonged lactation
43. Is increased in users of continuous combined HRT

HIV infection

44. In the UK 200 babies are born each year to women infected with HIV
45. About 20% of babies born to women infected with HIV are themselves infected
46. Over half of HIV infected women in London are known to their obstetricians at the time of delivery
47. Breastfeeding doubles the risk of HIV transmission in HIV infected women
48. There is evidence that Caesarean delivery reduces the risk of the vertical transmission of HIV
49. The prevalence of HIV infection world-wide is 1/1000 adult population
50. Over 70% of HIV positive adults are thought to be women

Colposuspension

51. Burch colposuspension for GSI has success rates up to 90% in the short-term
52. Is a first line management for a woman with predominantly stress symptoms
53. Has lower complication rates than vaginal operations
54. Can lead to detrusor instability
55. Can lead to worsening detrusor instability
56. Is associated with a 20% incidence of urinary retention postoperatively
57. Should be performed using a supra pubic catheter in order to keep the bladder empty during the operation
58. Is associated with increased risk of rectocoele postoperatively
59. May cause the occurrence of a cystocoele

Chorioamnionitis

60. Anaerobic infection is characteristic
61. Cannot occur in the presence of intact membranes
62. Should be immediately delivered by Caesarean section

Thyrotoxicosis in pregnancy and the neonate

63. Propyl-thiouracil is safe during breast feeding
64. Neonatal thyrotoxicosis does not occur if the mother is euthyroid
65. Neonatal thyrotoxicosis is normally apparent within 24 hours of birth
66. Neonatal thyrotoxicosis is reversible

Vaginal carcinomas

67. Are most commonly secondary tumours
68. Constitute less than 0.1% of genital tract malignances
69. The peak incidence is in the fourth and fifth decades
70. The minority are squamous

In normal spontaneous labour

71. Artificial rupture of membranes shortens the length of first stage
72. 50% of women will rupture membranes spontaneously by 4 cm dilatation
73. Moulding of the fetal head implies cephalopelvic disproportion
74. Contraction strength is stronger in multiparous women
75. Cardiotocography has reduced intrapartum fetal loss
76. Endogenous oxytocin plays an early role

Painful bleeding from the anus is a recognized feature of

77. Prolapsed rectum
78. Anal fissure
79. Endometriosis coli
80. Perianal haematoma
81. Recto-vaginal fistula

Regarding barrier methods of contraception

82. They reduce the risk of transmission of herpes simplex infection
83. Use of the diaphragm is associated with an increased risk of male urinary tract infections
84. They reduce the risk of cross infection from the bacteria chlamydia
85. The advantages of latex barrier contraceptives over the polyurethane ones is that the second is easily destroyed by oil-based lubricants
86. They reduce the risk of transmission of hepatitis A, B, HIV and Neisseria infections during vaginal intercourse

Jaundice appearing on the third day and still present at 2 weeks of age may be due to

87. Haemolytic disease of the newborn due to Rhesus incompatibility
88. Galactosaemia
89. Atresia of the bile duct
90. Phenylketonuria
91. Neonatal hyperthyroidism
92. Neonatal hypothyroidism
93. TORCH infection

Phaeochromocytoma in pregnancy

94. Characteristically presents under 20 years of age
95. May produce paroxysms of hypertension
96. May secrete dopamine
97. Causes a high output of 5-hydroxyindoleacetic acid in the urine
98. Is a recognized cause of impaired glucose tolerance

Regarding sexual function

99. Intact cognitive process is important for normal sexual function
100. Orgasm in the female partner is not necessary for fertilization to occur
101. 30% of women in their thirties are anorgasmic
102. Orgasmic dysfunction means sexual dysfunction
103. Intensive sexual counselling can improve sexual function in 90% of women
104. The commonest type of female sexual dysfunction is vaginismus
105. Dyspareunia can lead to sexual dysfunction
106. Sexual function can be improved by using vaginal lubricating creams

Acute inversion of the uterus

107. Is associated with preterm delivery
108. Is a recognized consequence of genital prolapse
109. Is more common in twin than singleton pregnancies
110. Is a recognized complication of ergometrine administration
111. Occurs more commonly when the placenta is sited in the fundus of the uterus
112. Is common after prolonged labour
113. Is treated by the hydrostatic method of O'Sullivan

Common causes of vaginal discharge in a prepubertal girl include

114. Ectopic ureter
115. *Neisseria gonorrhoae*
116. *Enterobius vermicularis*
117. Foreign body
118. Ovarian dysgerminoma
119. Candidiasis

Following PID there is an increased risk of

120. Hysterectomy
121. Ectopic pregnancy

Gestational trophoblastic tumours

122. Can occur following a normal delivery
123. Are always choriocarcinoma after a full-term pregnancy
124. May occur after an ectopic pregnancy
125. May also secrete oestrogens and progesterones
126. Secrete multiple forms of hCG
127. May present with persistent post-partum haemorrhage

Placental abruption

128. Is associated with a perinatal mortality rate of 9/1000 births
129. Has a recurrence rate of 16%
130. Is associated with cocaine use
131. When associated with premature labour should be treated with tocolytics
132. Can reliably be excluded by an ultrasound scan
133. If confirmed, expectant management is contraindicated
134. If large, is an indication for Caesarean section
135. Could lead to an increased level of D-dimers in blood
136. The amount of vaginal blood loss should be used as a guide for the estimation of the degree of abruption

The following are elevated in women with polycystic ovarian disease

137. Serum FSH
138. Serum TRH
139. Serum 17-hydroxyprogesterone
140. Serum oestradiol
141. Serum androstendione

Perinatal death

142. Congenital abnormalities account for 20% of all causes
143. Unexplained deaths in neonates over 2500 g account for 40% of cases

Peri-operative complications

144. Hypovolaemic shock may be the first manifestation of concealed post-operative bleeding
145. Postoperative internal bleeding may manifest with progressive anaemia
146. Pyrexia in the postoperative period may be a sign of an ileus
147. Pyrexia in the postoperative period may be a sign of haematoma
148. Pyrexia in the postoperative period may be associated with venous thrombosis
149. Once a vaginal vault haematoma has occurred it should be drained surgically

The biophysical profile

150. The disadvantage of this test is that it only measures indices of chronic fetal hypoxia
151. The use of this test can reduce perinatal mortality by over 10 times in high risk pregnancies
152. Correlates closely with fetal umbilical cord blood pH
153. An amniotic fluid pocket depth of less than 8 cm late in the third trimester indicates chronic fetal hypoxia
154. Perinatal mortality exceeds 80/1000 when BPP is less than four
155. Biophysical profile has a higher specificity than the non-stress test

Late complications of radiotherapy include

156. Leukopenia
157. Erythema
158. Bladder fibrosis
159. Vaginal stenosis

Radiological tests in pregnancy

160. Fetal weight estimations via ultrasound are more accurate when the fetal weight is around 3500–4500 g
161. The radiation dose of CT pelvimetry is higher than with X-ray pelvimetry
162. The dose of radiation to which the women is exposed during a venogram is higher than the dose of radiation at pelvimetry
163. Ventilation/perfusion scan exposes the patient to a higher dose of radiation than X-ray pelvimetry

Cervical cancer and pregnancy

164. Treatment should not be deferred as this worsens the prognosis
165. In early pregnancy cervical cancer is better treated by termination of pregnancy and radical surgery or radiotherapy
166. Vaginal delivery promotes direct spread
167. If diagnosed in late pregnancy a Caesarean Wertheim's hysterectomy should be performed or Caesarean section should be followed by radiotherapy after achieving fetal maturity at 36 weeks

Which of the following are true of Fallopian tube tumours?

168. The commonest are papillary adenosarcomas
169. May be suggested clinically by a watery vaginal discharge
170. May be suggested hystologically on a cervical smear
171. Surgery is the optimum treatment
172. Adjuvant chemotherapy may have a role

Cardiac disease and maternal mortality

173. The mortality from myocardial infarction is higher in the puerperium compared with early pregnancy
174. In the early 1990s substandard care was documented in the majority of cases of death associated with cardiac disease
175. Mortality in women with Eisenmenger's syndrome approximates 100% when pregnancy is continued to term
176. In women with Eisenmenger's syndrome termination of pregnancy does not offer significant improvement in survival rates over continuation of pregnancy
177. Fallot's tetralogy is associated with mortality rates of over 40%

The following associations are correct

178. Marcain — Fetal distress
179. Heparin — Two different types of thrombocytopenia
180. Syntocinon — Hypertensive crisis
181. Syntometrine — Cardiac arrest
182. Warfarin — 5% risk of fetal chondrodysplasia
183. Chloramphenicol — Neonatal haemolysis
184. Sulphonamides — 'Grey baby' syndrome
185. Anticonvulsants — Fetal neural tube defects
186. Nitrous oxide — Megaloblastic anaemia
187. Metronidazole — Oculogyric crisis

Minimal access surgery

188. Is a cost effective alternative to laparotomy
189. Requires less postoperative analgesia than vaginal surgery
190. If visceral damage occurs during laparoscopic surgery, laparotomy is indicated
191. Laparoscopically assisted vaginal hysterectomy is associated with lower intra-operative blood loss than open abdominal surgery

Urge incontinence

192. This is an involuntary loss of urine preceded by a sudden strong desire to void
193. Symptoms of stress, urge, urgency and frequency are highly specific for urge incontinence
194. Pelvic floor exercises are an effective form of treatment
195. Detrusor instability can only be diagnosed if cystometry shows an intravesical pressure rise > 15 cm H_2O at filling or on provocation
196. Increased trabeculation of the bladder on cystoscopy could be a sign of detrusor instability

Epidural analgesia

197. Is associated with long-term backache
198. Is relatively contraindicated within 12 hours of administration of low molecular weight heparin
199. Previous Caesarean delivery is a contraindication
200. Cardiorespiratory collapse is a known complication
201. Mendelson's syndrome is a known complication
202. Reduces pelvic floor muscle tone
203. Solely should be used for the treatment of hypertension in labour

Regarding complications of IUCDs

204. Absent threads suggest expulsion or perforation
205. Absent threads are an indication for hysteroscopy
206. The commonest reason for an intrauterine pregnancy is partial expulsion of the coil
207. The incidence of expulsion is $1/1000$ insertions
208. The incidence of PID in IUCD users after 20 days of insertion equals the background incidence for the population

Amniocentesis assists in the diagnosis of

209. Tay–Sach's disease
210. Cystic fibrosis
211. Rhesus allo-immunization

Conditions associated with ulcerative vulval lesions include

212. Behcet's syndrome
213. Ulcerative colitis
214. Herpes simplex
215. Chancroid

Forty patients participated in a randomized controlled trial of complete bed rest versus ambulation in the management of proteinuric hypertension in pregnancy. The measurement of urinary oestriol (mmol/l) in the two groups was as follows

	Rested group (n = 20)	Ambulatory group (n = 20)
Mean	52.1	365.6
SD	270.3	197.1
Range	180–1200	115–860

t = 2.08   Difference between means = 155.7   p = 0.022

The following statements are true

216. The standard error of the mean for the 'rested' group was 270.3
217. Patients were allocated alternately to 'ambulant' and 'rested' groups
218. The observed differences did not occur by chance
219. The value 't' refers to a test for the difference between the means
220. In the ambulant group 95% of the oestriol values were between 365.6 $+/-197.1$

HRT is always contraindicated with

221. Recent history of breast cancer
222. Previous endometrial cancer
223. Previous DVT
224. Surgery
225. Diabetes mellitus

A single Barr body is found in association with

226. Klinefelter's syndrome
227. Down's syndrome male
228. Turner's syndrome
229. Pituitary hypoplasia
230. Adrenogenital syndrome
231. Testicular feminization syndrome
232. Male with 21-hydroxylase deficiency
233. Superfemale

Which of the following gastrointestinal associations are true?

234. Diverticulitis	Intestinal fistula
235. Ulcerative colitis	Radiologically detected 'skip lesions'
236. Crohn's disease	Right sided hydronephrosis
237. Paralytic ileus	Hypokalaemia
238. Prevention of colonic carcinoma	HRT

Achondroplasia

239. Can be excluded by a normal femur length at 18 weeks scan
240. Is the most common lethal anomaly
241. Survivors are usually infertile
242. Inheritance is autosomal recessive
243. Causes mental retardation
244. Can be diagnosed by amniocentesis

The following are true associations

245. Abnormally high FSH level in the follicular phase of the menstrual cycle is associated with an increased risk of spontaneous miscarriage
246. Activated protein C resistance is associated with an increased risk of recurrent miscarriage
247. Women on immunosuppressive therapy have an increased incidence of spontaneous miscarriage

The following placentally transmitted infections that harm the fetus may be linked

248. Cheddar cheese   *Listeria monocytogenes*
249. Sheep faeces   *Toxoplasma gondii*
250. Oysters   Hepatitis A
251. Milking cows   *Chlamydia psittaci*

Magnesium sulphate

252. Causes respiratory depression before loss of deep tendon reflexes
253. Is proven to prevent eclamptic fits in pre-eclamptic women
254. Is excreted by the kidney, so doses must be reduced in women with protinuric hypertension
255. May cause diplopia, slurred speech and feelings of warmth
256. Overdose is treated with calcium carbonate

The following features are found in idiopathic hirsutism

257. Increased FSH secretion
258. Decreased SHBG
259. Dexamethasone suppresses renal function
260. Idiopathic hirsutism may be treated successfully by the oral contraceptive pill
261. Idiopathic hirsutism may be treated with the loop diuretic spironolactone
262. Plasma testosterone > 4 µmol / l

Rubella

263. Infection occurring early in the second trimester has a less than 1% risk of neonatal rubella syndrome
264. Once diagnosed immediate treatment with immunoglobulin reduces the risk of congenital malformation
265. The rubella haemagglutination inhibition test becomes positive within 4 days of the infection
266. Viraemia precedes the rash
267. Conjunctivitis is a characteristic feature

Hyperprolactinaemia

268. Carbergoline has fewer side effects than bromocriptine
269. Bromocriptine may cause renal failure
270. Surgery is advocated for pituitary tumours with frontal lobe extension

Regarding ovarian cysts

271. A 4 cm endometrioma can be successfully treated with GnRH analogues
272. They are present in 6% of asymptomatic women
273. Functional cysts are more likely to regress in younger women
274. The risk of ovarian cysts being malignant in premenopausal women is about 2%
275. Ovarian cysts can be confirmed to be benign if CA 125 levels are normal
276. Ovarian cysts often develop as luteinized unruptured follicles which occur in about 10% of cycles in infertile couples

Diagnostic amniocentesis at 16 weeks gestation is associated with an increased incidence of

277. Preterm labour
278. Talipes equinovarous

The umbilical cord

279. Contains nerves
280. Contains lymphatics
281. Vellamentous insertion is associated with congenital abnormality of the fetus
282. Fetal abnormalities are found in 40% cases of single umbilical artery
283. Umbilical artery blood flow is a reliable predictor of fetal distress
284. During cordocentesis, the transplacental approach is usually preferred with an anterior placenta
285. Chances of cord prolapse increase greatly if the length is more than 35 cm

A 25-year-old smoker at 32 weeks is found to have a growth-retarded baby on one scan. Which of the following may be associated with these findings?

286. Increased fetal plasma viscosity
287. A decrease in placental production of thromboxane and prostacyclin
288. Ingestion of more than 120 g alcohol daily
289. Essential hypertension
290. Oligohydramnios

and what would you do if a subsequent Doppler showed reversed end-diastolic flow?

291. Deliver immediately
292. Give steroids and then deliver immediately

Breastfeeding

293. Is associated with less than a 2% chance of pregnancy if the woman is amenorrhoeic

Dysfunctional uterine bleeding

294. Mefenamic acid reduces mean blood loss by 10%
295. In the short term hysteroscopic treatment is superior to hysterectomy
296. TCRE is safer than ELA
297. Progestins are more effective than danazol in endometrial preparation for a TCRE/ ELA
298. Tranexamic acid reduces mean blood loss by over 50%

PID

299. Chlamydia have been isolated in over 50% of cases of PID in the UK
300. Neisseria can be isolated in about 15% of cases of PID in the UK

ANSWERS TO PAPER THREE

The numbers of the correct answers are given

Sickle cell disease in pregnancy
3, 5, 6, 9, 10, 11
Sickle cell disease is characterized by the formation of an abnormal globin molecule (substitution of valine for glutamic acid residue at amino acid 6 position of the beta-globin chain). In the UK, sickle cell crisis occurs in 35% of affected pregnant women and is associated with 1–2% maternal mortality and a 4–6 times increase in perinatal mortality. Miscarriage, late fetal loss, type 2 IUGR, proteinuric hypertension, sepsis and thrombo-embolism are known complications. The use of heparin in prophylactic doses should be considered if the risk of thrombo-embolism is unacceptably high. Epidural is preferred because of a lower risk of hypotension. Antenatal diagnosis is currently available via CVS, amniocentesis and cordocentesis and recombinant DNA techniques. The IUCD is associated with a theoretical risk of infection and crisis. The POP is recommended.

Reference
Howard RJ, Tuck SM. Sickle cell disease and pregnancy. *Current Obstetrics and Gynaecology,* 1995; **5**: 36–40.

Colposcopy
13, 14, 15   (Premalignant disease of the cervix)
Colposcopic features of intraepithelial neoplasia are not necessarily present with HPV infection. The 'Schiller test negative' is synonymous with positive iodine staining. With increasing severity of intra-epithelial neoplasia the punctuation becomes coarser. Aceto-white staining may be present without immature squamous metaplasia, but with increasing immaturity aceto-white staining becomes more intense. Colposcopy is much less effective for the diagnosis of VIN than for CIN.

Reference
Shafi MI. Controversies in colposcopy. *British Journal of Hospital Medicine*, 1997; **58**: 246–247.

Match
21, 22
Neogest is a progesterone-only preparation. Femodene contains half the dose of gestodene stated.

Reference
Mims. October 1996, 298.

Primary pruritus vulvae

29   (Pruritus vulvae)

Primary pruritus vulvae is commoner in older women. It has no apparent primary cause and does not generally involve the anal area. Itching does not improve at night and when prolonged it could lead to depression and suicidal thoughts. Vulval skin biopsy is unnecessary unless a premalignant condition or malignancy is suspected.

References

Evans S. Vulval skin disease and the gynaecologist. *British Journal of Hospital Medicine*, 1997; **57**: 579–581.

Iffland C, Marwood R. Gynaecological aspects of vulval disease. Obstetrics and gynaecology. In: *Maternal and Child Health*. 1996; May: 130–135.

Maclean AB. Precursors of vulval cancers. *Current Obstetrics and Gynaecology*, 1993; **3**: 149–156.

Sarhanis P, Blackett AD, Sharp F. Intraepithelial neoplasia of the anogenital area: a multicentric condition. *Current Obstetrics and Gynaecology*, 1996; **6**: 92–97.

The Confidential Enquiries into Maternal Deaths in the United Kingdom (1991–93) reported that

32, 34   (The Confidential Enquiries into Maternal Deaths in the United Kingdom (1991–93))

The mortality from Caesarean section was 0.39/1000 (103 in total). Use of antacids cannot protect from Mendelson's syndrome. Only 40% of deaths from amniotic fluid embolism occurred before delivery. Avoidable factors were present in 85% of anaesthetic deaths. Eight women died from PPH compared to seven from APH.

Reference

Report on Confidential Enquiries into Maternal Deaths in the United Kingdom, 1991–1993. London: HMSO, 1996.

The risk of an endometrial cancer

36, 37, 38, 39, 41, 42   (Uterine tumours)

The risk of developing endometrial cancer is affected by a number of factors. The risk is increased 7.5 times in Tamoxifen users, is doubled if menarche has occurred before 12 years and in diabetic patients. It is also increased in nulliparous, obese and hypertensive women and those with hyper-oestrogenic conditions. Prolonged lactation with increased parity are protective factors as is use of combined oral contraceptives and continuous combined HRT. The incidence of an endometrial cancer in smokers is 10–30% lower than in non-smokers.

References

Lawton FG. Early endometrial carcinoma—no more TAH, BSO and cuff. In: Studd J, ed. *Progress in Obstetrics and Gynaecology*. Volume 10. Edinburgh: Churchill Livingstone, 1993; 403–413.

Lawton F. The management of endometrial cancer. *British Journal of Obstetrics and Gynaecology*, 1997; **104**: 127–134.

Rose P. Endometrial carcinoma. *The New England Journal of Medicine*, 1996; **335**: 640–648.

Semple D. Endometrial cancer. *British Journal of Hospital Medicine*, 1997; **57**: 260–262.

HIV infection
44, 45, 47, 48
The prevalence of HIV infection around the world is 1:250. Around 40% of the affected population are women. The incidence of HIV positivity varies among countries and urban and rural population. Only 16% of HIV positive women in London are known to care givers at the time of delivery. Caesarean section reduces the risk of transmission of HIV infection to the baby by 50%.

References

Johnstone FD. HIV and pregnancy. *British Journal of Obstetrics and Gynaecology*, 1996; **103**: 1184–1190.

Mercey D, Nicoll A. We should routinely offer HIV screening in pregnancy. *British Journal of Obstetrics and Gynaecology*, 1998; **105**: 249–251.

Newell M-L, Peckham CS. HIV-1 infection in pregnancy. RCOG PACE review. 96/05.

Olaitan A, Johnson M. Gynaecological problems in women infected with HIV. *Current Obstetrics and Gynaecology*, 1994; **4**: 189–192.

Colposuspension
51, 54, 55, 56   (Urinary incontinence: urodynamics)
The diagnosis of GSI should not be presumed in all patients with predominantly stress incontinence symptoms. The first line of management in such a patient is urodynamic assessment and/or non-surgical methods where appropriate. After this colposuspension should be considered for GSI. A urethral catheter is needed during this operation, with an inflated balloon in order to ensure correct placement of stitches and adequate bladder neck elevation. This operation has high success rate, but also a high incidence of complications, such as enterocoele, urinary retention, *de novo* detrusor instability. This operation can cure a cystocoele.

References

Cardozo L, Hill S. Urinary incontinence. RCOG PACE review 96/09.

Eckford SD, Keane D. Surgical treatment of urinary stress incontinence. *British Journal of Hospital Medicine*, 1992; **48**: 308–313.

Hilton P. The Stamey procedure for stress incontinence. *Current Obstetrics and Gynaecology*, 1991; **1**: 103–108.

Monga AK, Stanton SL. The Burch colposuspension. *Current Obstetrics and Gynaecology*, 1994; **4**: 210–214.

Chorioamnionitis
60
It can occur with intact membranes. Vaginal delivery is the preferred method.

Reference

Divers M. Infection and preterm labour, RCOG PACE, review 95/12.

Thyrotoxicosis in pregnancy and the neonate
66   (Thyroid and pregnancy)
Breastfeeding is contraindicated with antithyroid drugs. Although rare, neonatal

thyrotoxicosis is caused by maternal thyroid-stimulating antibodies (IgG) which readily cross the placenta. If they are in sufficient quantities they may stimulate the baby's thyroid making it thyrotoxic. These antibodies can be present in women with a history of Grave's disease who may be hypo or euthyroid at the time. Following birth, neonatal thyrotoxicosis may be apparent immediately (untreated women), but it is more likely to be delayed for a few days (the effect of maternal antithyroid drugs) or weeks (transplacental immunoglobulins initially block the thyroid-stimulating antibodies before they are broken down). Neonatal thyrotoxicosis is transient and normally regresses in 2–6 months as the antibodies are broken down.

Reference
Ritchie JKW. Diabetes and other endocrine diseases complicating pregnancy. In: Whitfield CR, ed. *Dewhurst's Textbook of Obstetrics and Gynaecology for Postgraduates*, 5th edn. Oxford: Blackwell Science, 1995; 262–276.

Vaginal carcinomas
67   (Vaginal tumours)
The peak incidence of the vaginal cancer is in sixth and seventh decades. They constitute 1–2% of genital tract malignancies, 90% are squamous.

In normal spontaneous labour
71   (Normal labour)
In the majority of women, the membranes remain intact at 4 cm dilatation. Moulding is a normal phenomenon of labour and does not necessarily mean cephalopelvic disproportion. Contraction strength is stronger in nulliparous women. Despite its widespread use, cardiotocography has not reduced intra-partum fetal loss. Prostaglandins play an early role in labour, oxytocin comes into action in the later part.

References
Beazley JM. Natural labour and its active management. In: Whitfield CR, ed. *Dewhurst's Textbook of Obstetrics and Gynaecology for Postgraduates*, 5th edn. Oxford: Blackwell Science, 1995; 293–311.
Care of the fetus during labour. In: Enkin MW, Keirse MJNC, Renfrew MJ, Neilson JP, eds. *A Guide to Effective Care in Pregnancy and Childbirth*, 2nd edn. Oxford: Oxford University Press, 1995; 207–220.

Painful bleeding from the anus is a recognized feature of
78, 79, 80
A prolapsed rectum is not usually associated with bleeding. Recto-vaginal fistulas are associated with faeculant vaginal discharge. If untreated perianal haematoma may rupture to discharge some clotted blood.

Reference
The rectum. The anus and anal canal. In: Mann CV, Russell RCG, ed. *Bailey & Love's Short Practice of Surgery*, 21st edn. London: Chapman & Hall Medical, 1992; 1215–1239, 1240–1275.

Regarding barrier methods of contraception

82   (Contraception and sterilization)

Use of the diaphragm is associated with an increased risk of female UTIs. Chlamydia is not a bacteria. Latex barrier contraceptives are easily destroyed by oil-based lubricants. Hepatitis A is transmitted via the oral-faecal route

Reference

Smith C. Barrier methods. In: *Contraception*. (Update Postgraduate Centre Series). Reed Healthcare Communications, 1995; 33–36.

Jaundice appearing on the third day and still present at 2 weeks of age may be due to

88, 89, 92   (Neonatology)

Neonatal jaundice appears within 24 hours in Rh-incompatibility and TORCH infection. Other causes are breast milk jaundice and neonatal hepatitis syndrome.

Reference

Jaundice in the newborn infant. In: Chamberlain GVP, ed. *Obstetrics by Ten Teachers*, 16th edn. Oxford: Edward Arnold, 1995; 318.

Phaeochromocytoma in pregnancy

95, 98   (Pre-eclampsia, eclampsia and phaeochromocytoma)

It is a rare cause of hypertension, diagnosed by history and examination (sweating, palpitation, paroxysmal hypertension), elevated urinary vanilyl mandellic acid, renal scan or MRI. Phaeochromocytomas secrete catecholamines. Surgical removal under alpha-adrenergic blockade is the treatment of choice.

Reference

Redman C. Hypertension in pregnancy. In: De Swiet M, ed. *Medical Disorders in Obstetrics Practice*, 2nd edn. Oxford: Blackwell Scientific Publications, 1990; 249–305.

Regarding sexual function

99, 100, 105, 106   (Sexual function)

Anorgasmia is not uncommon in women. About 10% of women in their thirties are anorgasmic. Orgasmic dysfunction and sexual dysfunction are not synonymous. Intensive counselling and education can improve sexual function in 65%. Frigidity is the commonest type of sexual dysfunction in women.

Acute inversion of the uterus

109, 111, 113

There is no direct relation with preterm delivery, genital prolapse or ergometrine administration. It is not common, but occurs more frequently after prolonged labour.

Reference

Beazley JM. Complications of the third stage of labour. In: Whitfield CR, ed. *Dewhurst's Textbook of Obstetrics and Gynaecology for Postgraduates*, 5th edn. Oxford: Blackwell Science, 1995; 368–376.

Common causes of vaginal discharge in a prepubertal girl
116 (Paediatric gynaecology)

Although all the other conditions (except ovarian dysgerminoma) can cause vaginal discharge they are uncommon causes. Threadworms (*Enterobius vermicularis*) are one of the commonest causes along with vulvitis and secondary vaginitis (due to poor hygeine) and amoebiasis. Other causes of discharge include systemic corticosteroid therapy (giving rise to candidiasis) and sarcoma botryoides.

Following PID there is an increased risk of
120, 121 (Pelvic inflammatory disease)

The increased risk of hysterectomy is eight times, that of an ectopic is seven times.

Reference
Joshi UY. Pelvic inflammatory disease. *Hospital Update*, February, 1993; 80–88.

Gestational trophoblastic tumours
122, 123, 124, 125, 126, 127 (Gestational trophoblastic disease)

Incidence following a normal delivery is 1 in 40 000–50 000.

Reference
Newlands ES. Trophoblastic disease. RCOG PACE review 96/10.

Placental abruption
128, 130, 135 (Antepartum haemorrhage)

Placental abruption has a recurrence rate of 6–10%. It is associated with cigarette smoking, cocaine use, pre-eclampsia and sudden uterine decompression. Its maternal complications include hypovolaemic shock (and associated coagulopathy), acute renal failure, and post-partum haemorrhage. Expectant management is acceptable if the fetal condition is satisfactory and greater maturity is to be achieved, but tocolytics are contraindicated. Ultrasound scan can easily miss out small abruptions or abruption of the posteriorly sited placenta and therefore should not be relied upon for diagnosis. Immediate delivery is necessary if signs of fetal compromise are present, but Caesarean section is not necessary if the fetus is dead. The revealed blood loss is a poor guide to the degree of placental abruption.

Reference
Roye JC, Malley RJ. Bleeding in late pregnancy. In: James DK, Steer PJ, Weiner CP, Gonik B. eds. *High Risk Pregnancy Management Options*. London: WB Saunders Company, 1994; 119–136.

The following are elevated in women with polycystic ovarian disease (PCOD)
141 (Polycystic ovarian disease [PCOD])

Levels of LH, testosterone, androstendione, oestrone are elevated. Levels of FSH, oestradiol, progesterone, 17-hydroxyprogesterone are reduced.

Perinatal death

142

The commonest cause of perinatal death is asphyxia, the second and third are congenital anomalies (20%) and prematurity (15%) respectively. In neonates weighing over 2500 g unexplained deaths constitute 10% of cases.

Reference

Stirrat GM. *Aids to Obstetrics and Gynaecology for MRCOG*, 4th edn. Edinburgh: Churchill Livingstone, 1997; 165–168.

Peri-operative complications

144, 145, 146, 147, 148   (Perioperative complications in obstetrics and gynaecology)

Spontaneous drainage of a vaginal vault haematoma is possible. Haematomas that are infected may give rise to a temperature.

The biophysical profile

151, 152, 155   (Biophysical profile – assessing the at risk fetus)

The major advantage of the biophysical profile is that it encompasses measurements of the markers of both acute and chronic fetal hypoxia. It is a highly reliable assessment of fetal well-being. The incidence of false negative result of biophysical scoring has been shown to be 0.8/1000, whilst the incidence of false negative result of non-stress test (CTG) is three per 1000. When less than four it is associated with a perinatal mortality more than 20 per 1000. Amniotic fluid pocket depth of 2–8 cm is normal.

Reference

Harman C, Menticoglan S, Manning F, Albar H, Morrison I. Prenatal fetal monitoring: Abnormalities of fetal behavior. In: James DK, Steer PJ, Weiner CP, Gonik B. eds. *High Risk Pregnancy Management Options*. London: WB Saunders Company, 1994; 693–734.

Late complications of radiotherapy include

158, 159   (Radiotherapy)

Leukopenia, erythropenia, thrombocytopenia and erythema are early complications of radiotherapy, whilst bladder fibrosis, vaginal stenosis and fistula formation are late complications.

Reference

Sproston ARM. Non-surgical treatment of cervical carcinoma. *British Journal of Hospital Medicine*, 1994; **52**: 30–34.

Radiological tests in pregnancy

Fetal weight estimation via ultrasound is less accurate at the extremes of weight. The radiation dose of CT pelvimetry (for a similar amount of information) is lower than that of X-ray pelvimetry. The radiation exposure at venogram is 0.5 rad vs. 0.5–1.1 rad at X-ray pelvimetry. The dose of radiation of a ventilation/perfusion scan is about one tenth of that of an X-ray pelvimetry.

Cervical cancer and pregnancy
165 (Cancer in pregnancy)
In general a delay in the treatment of cervical cancer in pregnancy adversely affects the prognosis. Thus it should be commenced as soon as possible, but due to the nature of treatment (fetal damage or potential loss of fertility) certain delays are acceptable. Vaginal delivery promotes vascular and lymphatic spread. When cancer is diagnosed in early pregnancy termination of pregnancy and surgery or radiotherapy are advisable. In late pregnancy delaying delivery by 1–2 weeks (until 28 weeks) could make significant differences to the fetal maturity which might be acceptable to the woman.

The following are true of Fallopian tube tumours
169, 171, 172 (Fallopian tubes)
The commonest are adenocarcinomas which can be suggested cytologically on a cervical smear.

Cardiac disease and maternal mortality
173 (Cardiac disease in pregnancy)
Myocardial infarction is associated with 40–50% mortality in the puerperium but rarely causes deaths in the first trimester. In the early 1990s, substandard care was documented in 27% of cases of maternal death associated with cardiac disease. In women with Eisenmenger's syndrome the mortality is 30–50% if the pregnancy is continued to term and 7% if terminated. Fallot's tetralogy is associated with mortality rates of 4–20%.

References
De Swiet M, ed. *Medical Disorders in Obstetric Practice.* Oxford: Blackwell Scientific Publications. 1994.
Oakley CM. Pregnancy and heart disease. *British Journal of Hospital Medicine*, 1996; **55**: 7: 423–426

The following associations are correct
179, 181, 182, 185, 186
Marcain is not known to be associated with fetal distress, though an epidural block can cause fetal heart decelerations. Heparin is associated with immediate-onset (i.e. non-idiosyncratic) thrombocytopenia, which has little clinical importance, and late onset (i.e. immunomediated) thrombocytopenia. Syntometrine is known to be associated with hypertensive crisis, syntocinon is not. Cardiac arrest is a rare complication of syntometrin when a high bolus dose is given. Sulphonamides used in late pregnancy are associated with neonatal haemolysis and chloramphenicol is associated with 'grey baby' syndrome. Continuous or repeat usage of nitrous oxide interferes with B12 metabolism and can cause megaloblastic anaemia. Metoclopramide is associated with oculogyric crisis.

Reference
British National Formulary, **35**; March 1998.

Minimal access surgery
188, 191 (Minimally invasive surgery)
Analgesic requirements are similar to vaginal surgery. Sometimes visceral damage can be repaired laparoscopically.

Urge incontinence
192, 195, 196   (Urinary incontinence: urodynamics)
The named or any other symptoms are non-specific. Pelvic floor exercises are for treatment of weakness of pelvic floor muscles associated with GSI.

References
Kelleher CJ, Cardozo LD. The conservative management of female urinary incontinence. *The Year Book of The RCOG 1994*. 123–135.
Cardozo LD, Hill S. Urinary incontinence. RCOG PACE review 96/09.
Richmond D. The incontinent women: 1. *British Journal of Hospital Medicine*, 1993; **50**: 418–423.
Richmond D. The incontinent women: 2. *British Journal of Hospital Medicine*, 1993; **50**: 490–492.

Epidural analgesia
198, 200, 202   (Analgesia/anesthesia in labour)
Epidurals are not associated with long-term back problems. An epidural can safely be used following a Caesarean section. Mendelson's syndrome is a known complication of general anaesthesia. Epidurals reduce the tone of the pelvic floor muscles and may be associated with an increased incidence of fetal head malrotation and instrumental delivery (not conclusive). They are associated with more frequent use of oxytocin in labour, but do not reduce its efficacy. Although they reduce peripheral resistance one should not rely exclusively on their anti-hypotensive effect and antihypertensive therapy should be administered in addition.

References
Collins RE, Morgan BM. Regional anaesthesia and obstetrics. *Current Obstetrics and Gynaecology*, 1995; **5**: 91–97.
Enkin M, Keirse MJNC, Renfrew M, Neilson J. *A Guide to Effective Care in Pregnancy and Childbirth*, 2nd edn. Oxford: Oxford University Press, 1995; 247–261.
Lewis M. Epidural and spinal anaesthesia in labour. *Current Obstetrics and Gynaecology*, 1996; **6**: 67–73.
Russell R, Reynolds F. Back pain, pregnancy, and childbirth. *BMJ*, 1997; **314**: 1062–1063.

Regarding complications of IUCD
206, 207, 208   (Contraception and sterilization)
Threads can be retracted into the uterine cavity whilst the IUCD remains *in situ*. They can effectively be detected by scan when normally sited.

References
Newton J. IUD safety and acceptability: recent advances. *Current Obstetrics and Gynaecology*, 1993; **3**: 28–36.
Newton J. Intrauterine contraceptive devices (IUCDs) and the levonorgestrel intrauterine system (IUS). In: *Contraception*. (Update Postgraduate Centre Series), Reed Healthcare Communications, 1995; 28–32.

Amniocentesis assists in the diagnosis of
209, 210   (Prenatal diagnosis)
It helps in monitoring rhesus allo-immunization, not diagnosing it.

Conditions associated with ulcerative vulval lesions include
212, 214, 215
Other associations are Crohn's disease and syphilis.

In a randomized controlled trial, the following statements are true
218, 219
The standard error of the mean is not the same as the standard deviation (standard error of the mean = SD/n). It was a randomized trial. Only 68% (1 SD) of the oestriol values were between 365.6 +/− 197.1 (95% values = 2 SD).

Reference
Swinscow TDV, Campbell MJ. *Statistics at Square One*, 8th edn. London: BMJ
   Publishing Group, 1996; 11–30, 52–85.

HRT is always contraindicated with
221   (Hormone replacement therapy)
There are some women with breast cancer who request HRT, many would argue that this is an absolute contraindication. Hypertension, PE, DVT and endometrial cancer are no longer considered to be contraindications. Surgery and diabetes mellitus are not contraindications.

A single Barr body is found in association with
226, 229, 230
Barr bodies occur in association with an inactive second X chromosome, which condenses into a heterochromatic mass. A male with Down's syndrome (47 XY) is most likely to have an extra chromosome 21, and will have only one X chromosome. Turner's syndrome (45 XO) has no inactive X chromosome. 47 XXY has one inactive X chromosome. A 'woman' with testicular feminization syndrome is genetically male (46 XY). A male with 21-hydroxylase deficiency has a normal genotype (46 XY). A superfemale (XXX) will have two Barr bodies.

Reference
Chromosomal basis of heredity. In: Thompson MW, McInnes RR, Willard HF, eds.
   Thompson & Thompson Genetic Medicine, 5th edn. Philadelphia: WB Saunders
   Company, 1991; 13–30.

Which of the following gastrointestinal associations are true?
234, 236, 237, 238
Fistula formation occurs in 5% cases of diverticulitis. 'Skip lesions' are a feature of Crohn's disease. The radiological features of ulcerative colitis are loss of haustration especially in the distal colon (earliest sign), ulceration, pseudopolyposis and pipe-stem colon (in chronic cases). A recent report in *The Lancet* suggests that HRT reduces the risk of colonic carcinoma.

Reference
Irving MH, Catchpole B. ABC of colorectal diseases. BMJ Publishing Group, 1992;

Achondroplasia
Achondroplasia is an autosomal dominant condition characterized by short extremities, which can be diagnosed by measuring femur length in the third trimester. It is neither lethal, nor it is associated with infertility or mental retardation.

Reference
Barr DGD, Goel KM. Disorders of bone and collagen. In: Campbell AGM, McIntosh N, eds. *Forfar and Arneil's Textbook of Paediatrics*, 4th edn, 1992; 1621–1691.

The following are true associations
246 (Abortion spontaneous/recurrent)
There may be an association with high LH levels in the follicular phase. There is no evidence to support the association with immunosuppressive therapy.

The following placentally transmitted infections that harm the fetus may be linked
Listeria monocytogenes is associated with soft cheese, pâté, undercooked chicken and hot dogs and prepared foods like coleslaw. *Toxoplasma gondii* can be transmitted indirectly by eating contaminated meat from sheep, cows and pigs. It can also be transmitted directly by contact with cat faeces. *Chlamydia psittaci* is associated with sheep and milking them. Oysters and raw shellfish are associated with hepatitis A but this does not affect the fetus.

Magnesium sulphate
255
Deep tendon reflexes are lost before respiratory depression occurs. It reduces the incidence of further fits in eclampsia (Collaborative Eclampsia Trial), but it has not yet been proved to be useful in preventing the first fit. It is excreted by the kidney and doses need to be reduced if renal function is poor (oliguria). Overdoses are treated with calcium gluconate.

Reference
Management of eclampsia. RCOG Guideline 10, 1996.

The following features are found in idiopathic hirsutism
258, 260, 262 (Hirsutism)
FSH secretion is unaffected. Dexamethasone suppresses adrenal function. The oral contraceptive pill increases SHBG therefore decreasing free androgens. Spironolactone acts on the distal tubule.

Rubella

266 (Infection in pregnancy)

Although the risks to the fetus are lower in the second trimester they are above 1% (6.4 at 4 months, 1.7 at 5 months). Immunoglobulin does not reduce the risk of congenital malformation, it is too late. The rubella haemagglutination test will become positive within 2 weeks of exposure. Viraemia and virus excretion precede clinical manifestations by 5–7 days. Other characteristics are arthralgia, lymphadenopathy and a mild pyrexial illness.

References

MacLean AB, Cockburn F. Maternal and perinatal infection. In: Whitfield CR, ed. *Dewhurst's Textbook of Obstetrics and Gynaecology for Postgraduates*, 5th edn. Oxford: Blackwell Science, 1995; 477–493.

Pastorek JG. Viral diseases. In: James DK, Steer PJ, Weiner CP, Gonik B, eds. *High Risk Pregnancy Management Options*. London: WB Saunders Company, 1994; 481–507.

Hyperprolactinaemia

268, 269, 270 (Hyperprolactinaemia)

Bromocriptine can cause retroperitoneal fibrosis, a rare cause of renal failure.

Regarding ovarian cysts

272, 273, 274, 276 (Ovarian tumours: epithelial)

GnRH analogues are ineffective for treating adhesions and large endometriomas (> 3 cm). Only 50% of women presenting with Stage One ovarian carcinoma have raised CA 125 levels.

Reference

Salat-Baroux J, Merviel PH, Kutten F. Management of ovarian cysts. *BMJ*, 1996; **313**: 1098.

Diagnostic amniocentesis at 16 weeks gestation is associated with an increased incidence of

277, 278 (Prenatal diagnosis)

Amniocentesis is associated with spontaneous abortions (0.5–1%), IUD, fetal respiratory difficulty at birth and allo-immunization, but not deep vein thrombosis, meconium ileus, cleft lip and cleft palate, and fetal heart rate alterations in late pregnancies.

Reference

Ramsay PA, Fisk NM. Amniocentesis. In: James DK, Steer PJ, Weiner CP, Gonik B, eds. *High Risk Pregnancy Management Options*. London: WB Saunders Company, 1994; 735–744.

The umbilical cord

282, 284

It contains two arteries and one vein, remnant of the yolk sac, Wharton's jelly and the allantois (occasionally). It absorbs water from the amniotic fluid. Vellamentous insertion is associated with vasa praevia and fetal haemorrhage, not fetal abnormality.

Umbilical artery blood flow is not reliable when predicting fetal distress. The umbilical cord is normally about 50 cm in length (7–180 cm range), cord prolapse is associated with polyhydramnios, footling breeches etc.

Reference
The placenta, cord and membranes. In: Chamberlain GVP ed. *Obstetrics by Ten Teachers*, 16th edn. Oxford: Edward Arnold, 1995; 7–14.

The following may be associated with IUGR
286, 288, 290, 292   (Intrauterine growth retardation)
It is hypothesized that the thromboxane:prostacyclin ratio in the placenta increases leading to vasoconstriction and platelet aggregation in the placental microvasculature, thereby reducing the blood flow to the fetus. IUGR is also associated with chromosomal abnormalities, pre-eclampsia (not normally essential hypertension), chronic maternal diseases, substance abuse, multiple pregnancy etc. Dopplers are only useful in growth retarded babies. Reversed end-diastolic flow is associated with a 25–40% mortality rate. Steroids should be given as they reduce the incidence of intra-ventricular haemorrhage within an hour but delaying delivery for the sake of lung maturity is not advisable.

References
Alcohol Consumption and Pregnancy. RCOG Guideline 9, 1996.
Beattie RB, Whittle MJ. The Management of IUGR. In: Bonnar J, ed. *Recent Advances in Obstetrics and Gynaecology, No 19*. Edinburgh: Churchill Livingstone, 1995; 35–44.
Pearce JM, Robinson G. Fetal growth and intrauterine growth retardation. In: Chamberlain G, ed. *Turnbull's Obstetrics*, 2nd edn. Edinburgh: Churchill Livingstone, 1995; 299–312.

Breastfeeding
293

Dysfunctional uterine bleeding
295, 298   (Menorrhagia – I)
Mefenamic acid reduces mean blood loss by 20%. Hysteroscopic treatment is superior to hysterectomy in terms of operative complications and postoperative recovery. ELA is safer than TCRE. Progestins are less effective than danazol or GnRH analogues in endometrial preparation.

Reference
Overton C, Hargreaves J, Maresh M. A national survey of the complications of endometrial destruction for menstrual disorders: the MISTLETOE study. *British Journal of Obstetrics and Gynaecology*, 1997; **104**: 1351–1359.

PID
299, 300   (Pelvic inflammatory disease)

PAPER FOUR

Allow 2 hours for completion of this paper

Features characteristically associated with haematocolpos in a 16-year-old girl include

1. Acute urinary retention
2. Failure of canalization of the Müllerian ducts
3. Persistence of the cloacal membrane
4. Primary infertility
5. Failure of fusion of the Müllerian ducts
6. Endometriosis
7. Co-existent developmental abnormalities of the mesonephric duct system
8. Closed spina bifida

The following characteristics match

9. Klinefelter's syndrome	Developmental failure of mesonephric duct
10. Testicular feminization	Developmental failure of urogenital sinus
11. Uterine agenesis	Developmental failure of Wolffian ducts
12. Hydatid cysts of Morgani	Paramesonephric remnants

Enterocoele

13. Can be congenital
14. Is a true hernia
15. Characteristically contains a loop of bowel
16. Is associated with dyschesia

Regarding azoospermia in men with normal FSH levels

17. Can be treated with corticosteroids
18. Can be treated with testosterone
19. Occurs with a germinal tubular defect of the testis
20. Is associated with absent vas deferens

Features of cytomegalovirus infection of the newborn include

21. Diffuse rash
22. Microcephaly
23. Asymptomatic
24. Diagnosis from a culture of urine sample
25. Hepatomegaly
26. Cataract

Serum changes suggestive of a premature menopause include

27. Elevated prolactin
28. Elevated LH
29. Low oestrone
30. Elevated androstenedione
31. Low 17-β oestradiol
32. Low FSH

Gestational hypertension

33. Plasma urate measurement is useful in the differential diagnosis
34. About 30% of pre-eclamptics are multiparous
35. Most cases of pre-eclampsia occur in the age group 16–19 years
36. The presence of twins increases the chance of eclampsia
37. Eclampsia is the main cause of maternal death

Ectopic pregnancy

38. Following a positive pregnancy test and an ultrasound scan showing an empty uterus a laparoscopy should be performed
39. Following laparoscopic linear salpingostomy, trophoblastic activity may continue in up to 20% of cases
40. Following conservative laparoscopic surgery the risk of a further ectopic is 15%
41. Following an ectopic pregnancy 15% will have another ectopic pregnancy
42. Following the diagnosis of an unruptured ectopic pregnancy antiprogestogens can be used for conservative therapy

A woman who is 12 weeks pregnant with a viable fetus is thought to have CIN III at colposcopy. A biopsy result revealed micro-invasive carcinoma. Treatment options include

43. Terminating the pregnancy and then treating the CIN
44. Performing a cone biopsy
45. Continuing with the pregnancy until viable (24 weeks), administering steroids and transferring to a unit with adequate neonatal facilities, performing a Caesarean hysterectomy

Spontaneous preterm labour has a recognized association with

46. Maternal hypertension
47. Previous cautery of the cervix
48. Previous cryosurgery to the cervix
49. Fetal oesophageal atresia
50. Bicornuate uterus
51. Chorioangioma of the placenta
52. Placental abruption
53. Raised maternal plasma AFP at 16 weeks and a normal fetus
54. Maternal hyperthyroidism
55. Asymptomatic bacteriuria

A 35-year-old nulliparous woman presents with anaemia secondary to menorrhagia. An ultrasound scan with saline suggests the presence of multiple 4–5 cm uterine leiomyomas, some intruding into the cavity. Which of the following options are appropriate for her management?

56. Commence GnRH analogues and operate after 9 months
57. Perform an emergency myomectomy
58. Transfuse and then send home on a prostaglandin synthetase inhibitor
59. Consider her for an endometrial resection/ablation
60. Consider her for laparoscopic myomectomy after GnRH analogues and HRT for 6 months
61. Consider her for embolization utilizing her right femoral vein

Match

62. Mifepristone   Shrinks fibroids
63. Depo-provera   Significant bone loss
64. HRT   Reduced incidence of colonic carcinoma
65. GnRH + HRT   Significant bone loss

ARDS

66. ARDS is associated with prolonged anaesthesia and large volume blood transfusion

With regard to closed laparoscopy (blind insertion of the Verres needle then trocar) the following statements are correct

67. Insertion of the Verres needle is associated with greater morbidity than the insertion of the trocar
68. Reported mortality rates are 4.09–77/100 000
69. The overall complication rate is 5.7/1000
70. Accredited gynaecologists cause more complications than trainees
71. The total incidence of visceral injury is 0.83/1000 of which 2.5% succumb
72. The total incidence of vascular injury is 0.75/1000 with a mortality rate of 0.8%
73. The lower mortality rate with vascular injury reflects its prompt diagnosis and treatment whereas 38% of visceral injuries are missed at the time of the procedure
74. The overall laparotomy rate for Verres needle injury is 3.9–4.2/1000 laparoscopies
75. The incidence of incisional hernia is 0.3%

Abnormally high concentrations of HCG in pregnancy are associated with

76. Fetal erythroblastosis
77. Anencephaly
78. Chorioangioma of the placenta
79. Carneous mole
80. Iniencephaly
81. Maternal alcoholism

Chronic pelvic pain

82. Accounts for 5% of gynaecological referrals
83. Post-coital aching, deep dyspareunia, pain of variable location and nature radiating through to the back suggests pelvic congestion syndrome
84. Pain occurring more than once a month, associated with abdominal distension and relieved by defaecation suggests endometriosis
85. If pelvic congestion exists GnRH agonists and add-back HRT are effective

The following are inherited as autosomal co-dominant trait

86. Rhesus group
87. Breast cancer

Chlamydia

88. 70% of affected women and 50% of affected men are asymptomatic
89. Incidence in UK is approximately 10/100 000
90. Adequate screening and treatment reduces the incidence of ectopic pregnancies

Recognized causes of cystic swelling of the breast include

91. Fibroadenosis
92. Ductal carcinoma
93. Hyperprolactinaemia
94. Degeneration within a colloid carcinoma
95. Dysgerminoma of the ovary
96. Granulosa cell tumour

A 23-year-old pregnant woman at 16 weeks has 2 + proteinuria. The following investigations should be carried out

97. 24-hour urine for protein estimation
98. Suprapubic aspiration of urine
99. Serum protein estimation
100. Renal scan
101. IVP

Ovarian hyperstimulation syndrome (OHSS)

102. Incidence is 4% following standard ovulation induction
103. When more than 30 oocytes are recovered there is a one in four chance of severe OHSS developing
104. Severe OHSS is characterized by ovaries greater than 15 cm diameter
105. May occur in one ovary
106. Is associated with an increased risk of venous thromboembolism
107. Can be prevented by giving pregnanediol immediately after oocyte recovery

Factors predisposing to maternal pulmonary aspiration of gastric contents during labour include

108. Decrease in gastric motility
109. The use of muscle relaxants
110. The effect of progesterone on the cardiac sphincter
111. The administration of oral magnesium trisillicate
112. Epidural analgesia

Intrahepatic cholestasis in pregnancy is characteristically associated with

113. Elevated total bile salts in the blood
114. Elevated plasma levels of the direct bilirubin fraction
115. Generalized pruritus in the absence of jaundice is the most common symptom
116. A positive direct Coomb's test in the neonate
117. Elevated serum acid phosphatase activity
118. Appearance in the third trimester
119. Racial variation
120. Neonatal jaundice

Associations of polycystic ovarian disease (PCOD) include

121. Loss of body hair
122. Failure of follicular maturation
123. Obesity
124. Insulin dependant diabetes mellitus
125. Adrenal hyperplasia
126. Hyperprolactinaemia

The following occur more frequently in pregnancy than in the non-pregnant state

127. Erythema nodosum
128. Carpal tunnel syndrome
129. Migraine
130. Cholestatic jaundice
131. Duodenal ulcer
132. Asthma
133. Pulmonary tuberculosis
134. SLE
135. Rheumatoid arthritis
136. Neurofibromatosis
137. Sarcoidosis

Ovarian cancer

138. The relative risks of developing ovarian cancer is 1%
139. If a woman carries the BRAC-1 gene her lifetime risk is almost 50%

Maternal oestrogen excretion during the last trimester of pregnancy is raised

140. With bed rest
141. By ampicillin therapy
142. In multiple pregnancy
143. By mandelic acid therapy
144. In rhesus sensitized pregnancy
145. In diabetes mellitus
146. In placental sulphatase deficiency
147. In adrenal hypoplasia
148. In renal agenesis
149. In sickle cell anaemia

With regard to miscarriage

150. Asherman's syndrome is a recognized complication of spontaneous miscarriage
151. Giving misoprostol then mifepristone 48 hours later has been shown to be 95% effective in managing miscarriages under 12 weeks
152. Incomplete abortion should not be managed with vaginal prostaglandins

Occipito-posterior position

153. Is common in anthropoid pelvis
154. Occipito-frontal is the presenting diameter
155. Accounts for 10–20% of vertex presentations in late pregnancy and early labour
156. Early rupture of membranes is common
157. About 90% rotate to occipito-anterior position as labour progresses
158. Persistent occipito-posterior should be delivered by Caesarean section

Regarding family planning

159. The progesterone only pill is as likely to fail as a copper coil
160. The condom is more effective than the diaphragm
161. Billing's method is similar to using the sponge when comparing failure rates
162. The levonorgestrel-releasing coil is as effective as Norplant in its first 2 years of use
163. Coitus interruptus is more effective than spermicides used alone
164. Male sterilization is less effective than female sterilization
165. Avoiding intercourse for 3–4 days around ovulation is a more reliable method of family planning than the progesterone only pill
166. Femidom (the female condom) is twice as strong as normal condoms

Nuchal translucency

167. Is diagnostic test for a chromosomal disorder

Cordocentesis

168. Prior fetoscopic localization of blood vessels is essential

Amniocentesis may be indicated

169. In diagnosing an intrauterine infection
170. At 36 weeks with rhesus-immunization

Side effects of the levonorgestrel releasing IUCD include

171. Acne
172. Hirsutism
173. Mastalgia
174. Breast atrophy
175. Mood changes

Match

176. Maternal renal cortical necrosis	Post-partum haemorrhage
177. Placental sulphatase deficiency	Fetal ichthyosis
178. Acute polyhydramnios	Dizygotic twins
179. Maternal serum alpha-fetoprotein >3 MOM	Gastroschisis
180. Raised maternal plasma factor VIII	Placental abruption
181. Pre-eclampsia	Sickle cell disease
182. Primary post-partum haemorrhage	Thrombocytopenic purpura
183. Eclampsia	Nephrotic syndrome

A geneticist's wife is very friendly with the man next door. The geneticist is concerned because he has noticed similarities between his son and the neighbour. He will be reassured if

184. Both his son and his neighbour are achondroplastic
185. Both his son and his neighbour have haemophilia
186. Both his son and his neighbour are A Rh positive
187. Both his son and his neighbour have testicular feminization syndrome
188. Both his son and his neighbour have Duchenne muscular dystrophy
189. The neighbour has cystic fibrosis
190. The neighbour has true Klinefelter's syndrome
191. The neighbour has beta-thalassaemia major
192. The neighbour has Down's syndrome
193. The neighbour has no children

Ritodrine

194. May cause hypokalaemia
195. Is less effective in ruptured membranes
196. Must not be used with steroids to stop preterm labour in diabetic patients
197. Has been shown to improve outcome on its own by prolonging pregnancy
198. The effective dose range is 150–350 µg/min
199. Has a negative chronotropic action on the heart
200. Causes peripheral vasodilatation
201. Can be used as a bolus to reverse uterine hypertonus

Causes of the largest pocket of amniotic fluid being greater than 7 cm include

202. Listeria infection
203. Normal pregnancy
204. Renal agenesis
205. Imperforate anus
206. Anencephaly
207. Iniencephaly
208. Hydrocephaly
209. Polycystic kidney

Regarding non-contraceptive effects of the combined oral contraceptive pill

210. It reduces menstrual loss in 20–30% of women
211. It reduces the incidence of PID by 50%
212. It increases the incidence of duodenal ulcers
213. It reduces the incidence of an ectopic pregnancy by 30%
214. It increases the incidence of fibroids by 17% after 5 years of use
215. It reduces the incidence of benign breast disease
216. It increases the incidence of myocardial infarction by 10 times in smokers
217. It increases the incidence of the breast cancer if used as a teenager
218. The increased risk of breast cancer is lifelong
219. The risk of venous thrombo-embolism with a non-gestodene containing pill is half that of a gestodene containing preparation (30 as opposed to 60/100 000 women)

The following pairs are characteristically linked

220. Neonatal convulsions   Hypercalcaemia
221. Hepatosplenomegaly   Galactosaemia
222. Polyhydramnios   Tracheo-oesophageal fistula
223. Neonatal cyanosis   Glucose-6-phosphate dehydrogenase deficiency
224. Blue sclera   Osteogenesis imperfecta

Amniotic fluid embolism

225. Is associated with artificial rupture of membranes
226. Is universally fatal
227. Maternal mortality due to amniotic fluid embolus has increased during last the two decades
228. In the early 1990s in the UK the majority of maternal deaths occurred due to substandard care

CIN

229. Takes 3–10 years to become carcinoma *in situ*

In iron deficiency anaemia

230. Depletion of iron stores is the earliest event to occur and the reduction of serum iron levels the latest
231. The drop in MCHC occurs before the fall in MCV
232. MCV is a better index of iron deficiency than haemoglobin concentration

Bacterial vaginosis

233. Is associated with a 10 times increased risk of preterm labour
234. Could be asymptomatic
235. Is associated with increased risk of infections after gynaecological surgery
236. Does not occur in virgins
237. The incidence is higher in women attending termination clinics than in those attending gynaecological outpatients' departments

Bleeding in pregnancy

238. Antepartum haemorrhage is defined as vaginal blood loss of more than 15 ml, prior to delivery of the fetus
239. One in 10 women will bleed at some point
240. Clotting abnormalities are known associations
241. Antepartum haemorrhage is associated with feto-maternal transfusion
242. 30% of all bleeding episodes in pregnancy occur in third trimester

Reversible impairment of spermatogenesis occurs with

243. Klinefelter's syndrome
244. Hypopituitarism
245. Alcohol intake
246. Sulphasalazine
247. Anabolic steroids
248. Acute pyelonephritis

External cephalic version (ECV)

249. Is most effective with an extended breech
250. Is contraindicated after the onset of labour
251. Is more likely to fail in nulliparous women
252. Is associated with preterm labour and uterine rupture

The incidence of cancer in pregnancy

253. The incidence of breast cancer in pregnancy is higher in the advanced age group
254. The prevalence of carcinoma of the cervix in pregnancy is around 5–10/10 000
255. Carcinoma of the vagina is extremely rare

Cardiac disease in pregnancy

256. The prevalence of cardiac disease in the Western world is 0.1%
257. Marfan's syndrome and Takayasu's syndrome are associated with coarctation of aorta and require delivery by Caesarean section
258. Palpitations are a common finding in pregnancy and usually do not require treatment
259. T wave inversion in lead III is a normal finding
260. Primary pulmonary hypertension is a contraindication to pregnancy

Urinary complications of gynaecological surgery

261. Unrecognized urinary tract trauma can present clinically similar to peritonitis
262. Urinary fistula may occur several weeks after gynaecological surgery
263. May present with an ileus

Fetal risks from a diabetic pregnancy include

264. Skeletal abnormalities
265. Cardiovascular abnormalities
266. Caudal regression syndrome with an incidence of 1/1000 diabetic pregnancies
267. Macrosomia
268. Symmetrical growth retardation
269. A 7% chance of major congenital anomalies

Chickenpox

270. Occurs in approximately 1 in 20 000 pregnancies
271. In the first trimester is associated with fetal varicella syndrome in 3%, and if it occurs late in pregnancy is associated with perinatal infection in up to 60%
272. Zoster immunoglobulin should be given if the maternal IgG levels are raised prior to delivery
273. Severe maternal infection should be treated with zidovudine
274. Is caused by a highly infectious DNA herpes virus, it can be prevented by using a live attenuated vaccine

Viral infection of the cervix

275. Human papilloma virus (HPV) types 16 and 18 are the RNA viruses most commonly associated with cervical cancer
276. Human papilloma virus infection can regress spontaneously
277. Viral infections involving the cervical squamous epithelium are only manifested by dyskaryosis

Spinal analgesia

278. Has a quicker onset of action than an epidural block
279. Is a technically more demanding procedure than an epidural block
280. Ideally should be widely used for pain relief in labour

Vulval cancer

281. Constitutes under 1% of all gynaecological malignancies
282. 2–3% of malignant tumours of the vulva are basal cell carcinomas
283. The squamous cell type is the commonest vulval cancer, constituting 50% of cases
284. Clinical staging is reliable
285. If less than 2 cm in diameter and with unilateral positive regional lymph node metastasis it is stage III disease
286. Spreads to the external iliac and obturator lymph nodes before involving deep and superficial inguinal and femoral nodes
287. Is associated with cervical cancer

Caesarean scar dehiscence

288. The incidence after a classical incision is 20–30%
289. The incidence after a lower segment uterine incision is less than 0.5%
290. The incidence after a De Lee incision equals that of a classical scar
291. Commonly presents with the clinical picture of massive internal bleeding
292. May occur before the onset of labour

Prognosis of endometrial cancer

293. 50% of endometrial cancers occur in the premenopausal age group
294. Five year survival rate stage for stage is similar to that of cervical cancer
295. Over 75% of women with endometrial cancer die of this disease
296. Adenoacanthoma of the endometrium has a very poor prognosis
297. Adverse prognostic factors include advanced age
298. Positive peritoneal cytology has no prognostic value

Hepatitis

299. HBsAg is the earliest marker of hepatitis infection

Cervical caps

300. Cannot be used in women with cervical dyskaryosis

ANSWERS TO PAPER FOUR

The numbers of the correct answers are given

Features characteristically associated with haematocolpos in a 16-year-old girl include
1, 2, 3, 6 (Abnormality of genital tract, Amenorrhoea, primary and secondary)
It is associated with primary amenorrhoea in girls with normal secondary sexual characteristics. It may arise because canalization of the fused Müllerian ducts fails to occur. Failure of fusion of the Müllerian ducts may result in double or bicornuate uteri. The uterus is derived from the paramesonephric duct, the mesonephric duct is unimportant in females and coexistent abnormalities are rare. There is no association with closed spina bifida. Other associations include reduplication of the metanephric duct.

The following characteristics match
12 (Abnormality of genital tract, Amenorrhoea, primary and secondary)
Klinefelter's syndrome is associated with testicular development and the development of the mesonephric duct (forming the prostate, seminal vesicle and ductules) but the testes do not function. In testicular feminization the urogenital sinus develops and may be thickened, there are absent tubes and ovaries but testes are present. The external genitalia fail to develop due to androgen insensitivity. Uterine agenesis is caused by failure of the development of Müllerian ducts.

Enterocoele
13, 14, 15 (Genital prolapse)
Dyschesia (difficulty in emptying the bowel) is associated with a rectocoele

Regarding azoospermia in men with normal FSH levels
20 (Male subfertility)
No medical treatment is of any use. A germinal tubular defect of the testis would be associated with raised FSH levels.

Features of cytomegalovirus infection of the newborn include
22, 23, 24, 25, 26 (Infection in pregnancy)
The rash is purpuric. Other associations include IUGR, intracerebral calcification, cerebral atrophy, seizures, psychomotor delay, learning disorders, expressive language delay, thrombocytopenia, haemolytic anaemia, splenomegaly, jaundice, deafness, chorioretinitis, optic atrophy, pneumonitis, dental abnormalities, long bone radiolucencies etc.

References
MacLean AB, Cockburn F. Maternal and perinatal infection. In: Whitfield CR, ed. *Dewhurst's Textbook of Obstetrics and Gynaecology for Postgraduates*, 5th edn, Oxford: Blackwell Science, 1995; 477–493.
Pastorek JG. Viral diseases. In: James DK, Steer PJ, Weiner CP, Gonik B, eds. *High Risk Pregnancy Management Options*. London: WB Saunders Company, 1994; 481–507.

Serum changes suggestive of a premature menopause include
28, 30, 31 (Menopause)
Oestrone and FSH levels increase. There is no change with prolactin levels.

Gestational hypertension
33, 34, 36 (Pre-eclampsia, eclampsia and phaeochromocytoma)
Most cases of pre-eclampsia occur in the age group 21–25 years. ARDS is the main cause of maternal death.

Reference
Redman C. Hypertension in pregnancy. In: De Swiet M, ed. *Medical Disorders in Obstetrics Practice*, 2nd edn. Oxford: Blackwell Scientific Publications 1990; 249–305.

Ectopic pregnancy
39, 41 (Ectopic pregnancy)
The woman might require a laparotomy, or this may be a complete miscarriage or a viable early pregnancy. Following conservative laparoscopic surgery the risk of a further ectopic pregnancy is 7%. Antiprogestogens have not been found to be useful, whereas methotrexate, potassium and prostaglandins have been used successfully.

Treatment options for a woman who is 12 weeks pregnant who is revealed to have a micro-invasive carcinoma
43, 45
A cone biopsy is not an option.

Spontaneous preterm labour has a recognized association with
49, 50, 51, 52, 53, 54, 55
Maternal hypertension is not associated with preterm labour, PIH is an important reason for iatrogenic prematurity. There is no evidence that cryosurgery, LLETZ or cautery increase the risk of preterm labour.

Appropriate management options for a 35-year-old woman with multiple uterine leiomyomas
(Fibroids)
Fibroid shrinkage (up to 49%) will occur after 3 months of GnRH therapy, further slight reductions may follow, thus surgery should be scheduled after 3 not 9 months. GnRH analogues alone should not be used for more than 6 months. There is no indication to perform an emergency myomectomy. Transfusion would be an option but prostaglandin synthetase inhibitors are unlikely to be of benefit in the long-term. Endometrial resection/ablation can be used to treat sub-mucus fibroids of 5 cm or under. Laparoscopic myomectomy would be an option in conjunction with resecting the sub-mucus fibroid. GnRH analogues are advised prior to laparoscopic treatment, giving them with HRT will not shrink the fibroids. Embolization would be an option but canulization utilizes the artery (not the vein).

Match

62, 64

Depo-provera is not associated with significant bone loss. GnRH + HRT prevents significant bone loss.

ARDS

66

With regard to closed laparoscopy the following statements are correct

68, 69, 70, 71, 72, 73, 74, 75   (Minimally-invasive surgery)

Insertion of the trocar is associated with greater morbidity than insertion of the Verres needle.

Abnormally high concentrations of HCG in pregnancy are associated with

76, 78

Other causes are multiple pregnancy, hydatidiform mole, wrong gestational age etc.

Reference

Davey DA. Normal pregnancy: anatomy, endocrinology and physiology. In: Whitfield CR, ed. *Dewhurst's Textbook of Obstetrics and Gynaecology for Postgraduates*, 5th edn. Oxford: Blackwell Science, 1995; 87–108.

Chronic pelvic pain

82, 83   (Chronic pelvic pain)

Pain occurring more than once a month, associated with abdominal distension and relieved by defaecation suggests irritable bowel syndrome. Medroxyprogesterone acetate may help but if pelvic congestion exists, GnRH agonists and add-back HRT are not effective.

Reference

William Stones R. Chronic pelvic pain. RCOG PACE review 97/01.

The following are inherited as autosomal co-dominant trait

86

There is some evidence to suggest that certain breast cancers may be inherited as autosomal dominant conditions. Other co-dominant traits include ABO, Kell, MNS blood groups, haptoglobin, HLA system, adenylate kinase and acid phosphatase.

Reference

Connor M, Ferguson-Smith M. *Medical Genetics*, 5th edn. Oxford: Blackwell Science, 1997; 69–81.

Chlamydia

88, 90

Incidence in UK is approximately 100/100 000

Reference

CMO's Expert Advisory Group on Chlamydia trachomatis. Department of Health, London.

Recognized causes of cystic swelling of the breast include
91, 94
Ductal carcinoma causes nipple discharge. Hyperprolactinaemia causes galactorrhoea. Other causes are papillary cystadenoma, galactocoele, serocystic disease of Brodie, lymphatic cyst etc.

Reference
The breast. In: Mann CV, Russell RCG, eds. *Bailey & Love's Short Practice of Surgery*, 21st edn. London: Chapman & Hall Medical, 1992; 788–821.

A 23-year-old pregnant woman at 16 weeks has 2+ proteinuria. The following investigations should be carried out
97, 99, 100   (Renal tract in pregnancy)
An MSSU is sufficient to rule out a UTI as a cause. An IVP is unnecessary, it is indicated for the investigation for recurrent UTIs and haematuria.

Reference
Davey DA. Hypertensive disorders of pregnancy. In: Whitfield CR, ed. *Dewhurst's Textbook of Obstetrics and Gynaecology for Postgraduates*, 5th edn. Oxford: Blackwell Science, 1995; 175–215.

Ovarian hyperstimulation syndrome (OHSS)
102, 103, 105, 106   (Infertility–II)
Severe OHSS is characterized by ovaries greater than 12 cm diameter. It may occur in one ovary (assisted reproductive techniques are used in women with just one ovary).

Reference
RCOG Guideline 5, January 1995

Factors predisposing to maternal pulmonary aspiration of gastric contents during labour include
108, 109, 110
Magnesium trisillicate reduces gastric acidity and does not predispose to aspiration of gastric contents. Epidural analgesia does not affect the cardiac sphincter.

References
Hospital practices. In: Enkin MW, Keirse MJNC, Renfrew MJ, Neilson JP, eds. *A Guide to Effective Care in Pregnancy and Childbirth*, 2nd edn. Oxford: Oxford University Press, 1995; 197–207.
Ritchie JWK. Obstetric operations and procedures. In: Whitfield CR, ed. *Dewhurst's Textbook of Obstetrics and Gynaecology for Postgraduates*, 5th edn. Oxford: Blackwell Science, 1995; 388–400.

Intrahepatic cholestasis in pregnancy is characteristically associated with
113, 114, 115, 118, 119
It usually appears in the third trimester, is characterized by generalized pruritus due to elevated bile salts in the blood as a consequence of intrahepatic cholestasis caused by raised oestrogen levels in the blood. It is more common in women of Asian origin. There is a positive family history in 44% of cases. It recurs in 45% cases. It is associated with preterm labour (59%), intrauterine death and post-partum haemorrhage (8–22%). It is not associated with a positive direct Coomb's test or neonatal jaundice. Serum alkaline phosphatase level is elevated.

References
Fagan EA. Disorders of the liver, biliary system and pancreas. In: De Swiet M, ed. *Medical Disorders in Obstetrics Practice*, 2nd edn. Oxford: Blackwell Scientific Publishers, University Press, 1994; 426–520.
Williamson C, Nelson-Piercy C. Liver disease in pregnancy. *British Journal of Hospital Medicine*, 1997, **58**(5): 213–216.

Associations of polycystic ovarian disease (PCOD) include
122, 123, 125, 126   (Polycystic ovarian disease [PCOD])
Failure of follicular maturation, hirsutism, obesity (25%), adrenal hyperplasia (10%), hyperprolactinaemia (15%) and insulin resistance (75%) leading to non-insulin-dependent diabetes mellitus are associated with PCOD.

The following occur more frequently in pregnancy than in the non-pregnant state
127, 128, 130, 134, 136

Reference
De Swiet M, ed. *Medical Disorders in Obstetrics Practice*, 2nd edn. Oxford: Blackwell Scientific Publications, 1994.

Ovarian cancer
138, 139   (Ovarian tumours: epithelial)

Reference
Eccles DM. Ovarian cancer genetics and screening for ovarian cancer. RCOG PACE review 97/06.

Maternal oestrogen excretion during the last trimester of pregnancy is raised
140, 142, 144, 145, 149
It is raised in cases of hyperplacentosis. It is decreased in placental sulphatase deficiency, adrenal hypoplasia, IUGR, acute pyelonephritis and therapy with antibiotics, aspirin and phenylbutazone.

References
Chard T, Macintosh MCM. Biochemical screening for Down's syndrome. In: Studd J, ed. *Progress in Obstetrics and Gynaecology*, Volume 11. Edinburgh: Churchill Livingstone, 1994; 39–52.

Davey DA. Normal pregnancy: anatomy, endocrinology and physiology. In: Whitfield CR, ed. *Dewhurst's Textbook of Obstetrics and Gynaecology for Postgraduates*, 5th edn. Oxford: Blackwell Science, 1995; 87–108.

With regard to miscarriage
(Abortion spontaneous/recurrent)
Asherman's syndrome is a complication of septic abortion and/or over-zealous curettage. Mifepristone is given before misoprostol. Vaginal prostaglandins are acceptable practice and could be safer alternatives to surgical evacuation

Occipito-posterior position
153, 154, 155, 156, 157   (Presentations and positions)
Vaginal delivery is preferred, unless difficult.

Reference
Ritchie JWK. Malpositions of the occiput and malpresentations. In: Whitfield CR, ed. *Dewhurst's Textbook of Obstetrics and Gynaecology for Postgraduates*, 5th edn. Oxford: Blackwell Science, 1995; 346–367.

Regarding family planning
159, 161, 162, 163, 166   (Contraception and sterilization)
User failure rates per 100 women years:

POP	1.2
Copper coil	0.3–4
Condom	3.6
Diaphragm	1.9
Billing's method	10–25
Sponge	9–25
LNG-IUCD	0.2
Norplant in its first 2 years of use	0.2
Coitus interruptus	6.7
Spermicides used alone	9–25
Male sterilization	0.02
Female sterilization	0.13
Sympto-thermal	3.6

Reference (for all contraceptive questions):
Guiellebaud J. *Contraception. Your Questions Answered*. Edinburgh: Churchill Livingstone, 1985.

Nuchal translucency
(Prenatal diagnosis)
Nuchal translucency is a screening test. It is neither diagnostic for chromosomal disorders nor is it associated with neural tube defects. In the absence of a chromosomal disorder it may be associated with congenital heart defects.

Cordocentesis
(Prenatal diagnosis)
Insertion of the cord in the placenta and blood vessels are localized with ultrasound.

Amniocentesis may be indicated
169 (Prenatal diagnosis)
It is only indicated in rhesus-immunization if the antibody titre is rising. Nowadays scans and cordocentesis are more readily used.

Side effects of the levonorgestrel-releasing IUCD include
171, 172, 173, 175 (Contraception and sterilization)
Progestogens promote glandular development in the breast.

Match
176, 177, 179, 181, 182 (Post-partum haemorrhage, Prenatal diagnosis)
Acute polyhydramnios is usually associated with monozygotic twins. Though the kidney may be affected in eclampsia, nephrotic syndrome is a different entity. Placental abruption leading to DIC will reduce the levels of factor VIII.

Reference
Rogers M, Barneston R StC. Diseases of the skin. In: Campbell AGM, McIntosh N, eds. *Forfar and Arneil's Textbook of Paediatrics*, 4th edn. Edinburgh: Churchill Livingstone, 1992; 1693–1727.

Geneticist's wife and neighbour
187, 189, 190, 192
The geneticist will only be reassured if the neighbour is infertile or dead. He may feel reassured about the X-linked conditions (haemophilia and Duchenne muscular dystrophy) but it does not rule out the neighbour as a father.

References
Neilson JP. Antenatal diagnosis of fetal abnormality and Whitfield CR. Blood Disorders in Pregnancy. In: Whitfield CR, ed. *Dewhurst's Textbook of Obstetrics and Gynaecology for Postgraduates*, 5th edn. Oxford: Blackwell Science, 1995; 221–239, 228–250.
Griffin JE, Wilson JD. Disorders of the testes and Mendell JR, Griggs RC. Inherited, metabolic, endocrine, and toxic myopathies. In: Isselbacher KJ, Braunwald E, Wilson JD, Martin JB, Fauci AS, Kasper DL, eds. *Harrison's Principles of Internal Medicine*, 13th edn. New York: McGraw-Hill, Inc., 1994; 2006–2017, 2383–2393.

Ritodrine
194, 195, 198, 200 (Premature labour)
It can be used in diabetic patients but blood glucose must be monitored closely, as both ritodrine and steroid increase it (insulin requirement may increase up to 30 times). The outcome improves because of enhanced lung maturity by the steroids. There is no evidence that prolonging pregnancy by ritodrine will have any further beneficial effects. It must not be used as a bolus dose because of its negative inotropic action and positive chronotropic action on the cardiovascular system.

References
Beta-agonists for the care of women in preterm labour. RCOG Guideline 1a, 1997.
Report on Confidential Enquiries into Maternal Deaths in the United Kingdom, 1991–1993. London: HMSO, 1996.

Causes of the largest pocket of amniotic fluid being greater than 7 cm include
202, 203, 205, 206, 207   (Polyhydramnios/oligohydramnios)
Seven centimetres is normal and not polyhydramnios. Polyhdramnios occurs when the greatest depth of amniotic fluid is over 8 cm. As the question asks for causes greater than 7 cm this includes the causes of polyhydramnios. Other causes include maternal diabetes, cardiac and renal disease, hydrops fetalis, multiple pregnancy (12%), fetal cardiac arrhythmia, severe deflexion of the fetal head (due to functional obstruction of the oesophagus), facial clefts and neck masses interfering with swallowing, duodenal and oesophageal atresia, achondroplasia, chorioangioma of the placenta etc.

Reference
Stark C. Disorders of the amniotic fluid. In: Frederickson HL, Wilkins-Haug L, eds. *Ob/Gyn Secrets*. Philadelphia: Hanley & Belfus Inc., 1991; 217–220.

Regarding non-contraceptive effects of the combined oral contraceptive pill
211, 215, 216, 217
It reduces menstrual loss in 60–80% of women. There is evidence that the incidence of duodenal ulcers is reduced. Ectopic pregnancies are reduced by 90%. The incidence of fibroids is reduced by 17% after 5 years of use. After 10 years of stopping the pill the risk of breast cancer is reduced to the background level. Although the first part of statement 219 is true, the figures are not. They should be 15 and 30 respectively (60 is the risk during pregnancy).

References
McPherson K. Third generation oral contraception and venous thromboembolism. *BMJ* 1996; **312**: 68–69.
Owen Drife J. *The Benefits and Risks of Oral Contraceptive Today*, 2nd edn. London: Parthenon Publishing Group; 1996.

The following pairs are characteristically linked
221, 222, 223, 224
Hypocalcaemia causes neonatal convulsions.

Reference
Cockburn F. Neonatal care for obstetricians. In: Whitfield CR, ed. *Dewhurst's Textbook of Obstetrics and Gynaecology for Postgraduates*, 5th edn. Oxford: Blackwell Science, 1995; 454–476.

Amniotic fluid embolism

225 (Amniotic fluid embolus)

Amniotic fluid embolism occurs with an incidence of 1/80 000 pregnancies. Maternal age more than 35 years, high parity, over distension of the uterus, use of syntocinon, intrauterine manipulations (e.g. artificial rupture of membranes), hypertonic uterine activity, and partial or complete rupture of the uterus are all risk factors. Maternal mortality due to amniotic fluid embolism has fallen slightly during last two decades but it is fatal more than 80% of the time. Substandard care has been documented in 20% of cases in the early 1990s.

References

Report on Confidential Enquiries into Maternal Deaths in the United Kingdom, 1991–1993. London: HMSO, 1996.

Still DR. Postpartum haemorrhage and other problems of the third stage. In: James DK, Steer PJ, Weiner CP, Gonik B. eds. *High Risk Pregnancy Management Options.* London: WB Saunders Company, 1994; 1167-1181.

CIN

229 (Premalignant disease of the cervix)

Reference

Anderson MC. The natural history of cervical intraepithelial neoplasia. *Current Obstetrics and Gynaecology.* 1991; 1: 124–129.

In iron deficiency anaemia

232 (Anaemia in pregnancy)

Iron deficiency first manifests with depletion of the iron stores. Reduction in haemoglobin concentration occurs last. Low red blood cell indices (MCV, MCH and MCHC) are helpful in the diagnosis. As iron deficiency anaemia develops the MCV falls first followed by a drop in MCHC and hypochromia occurs. The drop in haemoglobin occurs after the reduction in serum iron levels.

Bacterial vaginosis

234, 235, 237

The risk of preterm labour in association with bacterial vaginosis is two and a half times increased. Bacterial vaginosis can occur in virgins, but the incidence is low.

References

Emens JM. Intractable vaginal discharge. *Current Obstetrics and Gynaecology,* 1993; 3: 41–47.

Lamont RF. Bacterial vaginosis. *The Year Book of the RCOG 1994,* 149–158.

Bleeding in pregnancy

240, 241 (Antepartum haemorrhage)

Bleeding before 24 weeks of pregnancy is a threatened miscarriage, therefore the definition should include 'after 24 weeks of gestation'. One in five women will bleed at some point in pregnancy and only 4% of all bleeding episodes occur in third trimester.

Reference

Neilson JP. Antepartum haemorrhage. In: CR Whitfield, ed. *Dewhurst's Textbook of Obstetrics and Gynaecology for Postgraduates*, Fifth edn. 1995; 164–174.

Reversible impairment of spermatogenesis occurs with
245, 246, 247, 248

Klinefelter's syndrome and hypopituitarism cause irreversible impairment. If excessive, alcohol intake can result in irreversible damage. Treatment of UTIs and pyelonephritis can affect sperm production.

Reference

Paul S. Infertility. In: Paul S, ed. *An Essential Book in Obstetrics and Gynaecology*, Vol. 1. Calcutta: Standard Book House, 1996; 126–153.

External cephalic version (ECV)
251, 252   (Breech)

Extended legs make ECV technically difficult and increase the risk of failure. ECV can be performed in early labour. It is associated with preterm labour and uterine rupture as well as cord accident, placental abruption and sensitization of a rhesus-negative woman.

References

Burr RW, Johanson RB. Breech presentation: is external cephalic version worthwhile? In: Studd J, ed. *Progress in Obstetrics and Gynaecology*, Volume 12, Edinburgh: Churchill Livingstone, 1996; 87–98.

Harrold A, Owen P. External cephalic version. *British Journal of Hospital Medicine*. 1997, **57**(4): 157–158.

The incidence of cancer in pregnancy
253, 254, 255   (Cancer in pregnancy)

Cardiac disease in pregnancy
258, 259, 260   (Cardiac disease in pregnancy)

The prevalence of cardiac disease in the Western world is estimated to be 1%. Marfan's syndrome is associated with dissecting aortic aneurysms. Takayasu's arteritis may cause narrowing of the vessels around the aortic arch and also aneurysmal dilatation. Uncorrected coarctation of the aorta should be delivered by Caesarean section, Marfan's do not automatically need a Caesarean. Palpitations and soft systolic heart murmur are common findings in pregnancy and are not necessarily indicative of cardiac disease.

Reference

Oakley, CM. Pregnancy and heart disease. *British Journal of Hospital Medicine*, 1996, **55**(7): 423–426.

Urinary complications of gynaecological surgery
261, 262, 263   (Perioperative complications)

Fetal risks from a diabetic pregnancy

264, 265, 266, 267, 268, 269   (Diabetes and pregnancy)

Asymmetrical growth retardation can also occur in a diabetic pregnancy if the diabetes is long-standing or associated with diabetic angiopathy.

Reference

London MB, Gaffe SG. Diabetes mellitus. In: James DK, Steer PJ, Weiner CP, Gonik B. eds. *High Risk Pregnancy Management Options.* London: WB Saunders Company, 1994; 277–297.

Chickenpox

271, 274

Occurs in approximately 1:2000 pregnancies. Zoster immunoglobulin should be given if the maternal IgM levels are raised prior to delivery. IgG is a marker of previous infection whereas IgM is a marker of recent infection. Acyclovir should be used to treat severe or progressive infections.

Reference

Gilbert GL. Chickenpox during pregnancy. *BMJ,* 1993; **306**: 1079–1080.

Viral infection of the cervix

276   (Premalignant disease of the cervix)

Papilloma viruses are DNA viruses. HPV type 16 and 18 as well as 31, 33 and 35 are found in over 90% of invasive cervical cancers. Dyskaryosis is one of the manifestations of viral infections of cervical epithelium. Others include invasive cancer and koilocytosis.

References

Blomfield PI. Wart virus and cervical cancer. *Current Obstetrics and Gynaecology,* 1991; **1**: 130–136

MacLean AB, Macnab FCM. The role of viruses in gynaecological oncology. In: Studd J, ed. *Progress in Obstetrics and Gynaecology,* Volume 12. 1996; 402–417.

Spinal analgesia

278   (Analgesia/anaesthesia in labour)

Spinal analgesia is easier to administer than an epidural. It has a quicker onset and shorter action than an epidural so it is not recommended for use in labour.

Reference

Lewis M. Epidural and spinal anaesthesia in labour. *Current Obstetrics and Gynaecology,* 1996; **6**: 67–73

Vulval cancer
282, 285, 287   (Vulva)
Vulval carcinoma constitutes 5% of all gynaecological malignancies. Squamous cell carcinoma is the commonest type constituting 80–90% of vulval cancers. Its clinical staging is very unreliable. Spread occurs first to the superficial and deep inguinal and femoral nodes, then to the external iliac and obturator nodes. 15–30% of women with vulval cancer have/will develop cervical cancer.

References
Evans S. Vulval skin disease and the gynaecologist. *British Journal of Hospital Medicine* 1997, **57**(11): 579–581.
Helm CW, Shingleton HM. The management of squamous cell carcinoma of the vulva. *Current Obstetrics and Gynaecology*, 1992; **2**: 31–37.

Caesarean scar dehiscence
289, 292   (Caesarean section)
The incidence of scar dehiscence after a previous classical incision is the highest at about 9%. A De Lee incision has a lower incidence of this complication and is advised if possible. The clinical picture of a massive haemorrhage at the dehiscence of the uterine scar is uncommon.

Prognosis of endometrial cancer
294, 297   (Uterine tumours)
Only 25% of cases occur in premenopausal age. About 25% of women affected by endometrial cancer die of this disease. Adenoacanthoma has a good prognosis. Positive peritoneal cytology has adverse prognostic value.

References
Irwin CJR. The management of endometrial carcinoma. *British Journal of Hospital Medicine*, 1996; **55**: 308–309.
Lawton FG. Early endometrial carcinoma – no more TAH, BSO and cuff. In: Studd J, ed. *Progress in Obstetrics and Gynaecology*, Volume 10. Edinburgh: Churchill Livingstone, 1993; 403–413.
Lawton F. The management of endometrial cancer. *British Journal of Obstetrics and Gynaecology*, 1997; **104**: 127–134.
Rose P. Endometrial carcinoma. *The New England Journal of Medicine*, 1996; **335**: 640–648.
Semple D. Endometrial cancer. *British Journal of Hospital Medicine*, 1997; **57**: 260–262.

Hepatitis
299

Cervical caps
Barrier methods protect against the development of cervical dyskaryosis.

PAPER FIVE

Allow 2 hours for completion of this paper

Norplant

1. Contains five rod-shape capsules for sub-dermal insertion
2. Initial plasma levels (day 1) are 10 times higher than at 6 months
3. Is associated with an increased risk of developing functional ovarian cysts
4. If inserted on the first day of the menstrual cycle does not require extra contraceptive cover
5. If inserted within 21 days of delivery does not require extra contraceptive cover
6. If inserted within 21 days of termination of pregnancy does not require extra contraceptive cover
7. Causes irregular vaginal bleeding in 60–100% of users in the first year
8. Failure rates differ with each year of use
9. It is the most successful, reversible, long-term contraceptive agent to date
10. Raised progestogen levels persists for 28 days after removal of implants

Currently the 5 year survival for patients with vulval cancer

11. In stage four disease is 20%
12. Is 75% if lymph nodes are not involved
13. Is 10% if lymph nodes are involved

Vulval skin

14. Is exquisitely sensitive to radiation

Amniotic fluid embolism may present with

15. Adult respiratory distress
16. Cardiovascular collapse
17. Haemorrhage
18. Sudden death

Methotrexate in the treatment of ectopic pregnancy

19. Is contraindicated if a fetal heart beat is seen outside the uterine cavity
20. Is accompanied by an immediate fall in serum beta HCG levels
21. Is successful in >90% of selected cases

Anaemia in pregnancy

22. Iron requirements are at their highest level in the late third trimester
23. Vitamin B12 deficiency is the commonest cause of megaloblastic anaemia
24. The overall incidence of megaloblastic anaemia in the UK is 5%

VIN

25. Presents with vulval itching
26. VIN associated cancers are commoner in young women
27. VIN has a malignant potential similar to CIN
28. The risk of progression of VIN to invasive cancer is greater in older women

TENS

29. Electrodes should be placed over the posterior rami of T10-L1 and S2-4
30. Works by stimulating large sensory fibres

Breech presentation

31. The incidence at 32 weeks gestation is 16%
32. The commonest type is the flexed breech
33. Is associated with handicap rates of 20% regardless of mode of delivery
34. Fetal weight estimation via ultrasound scan in late third trimester is more useful than X-ray pelvimetry in deciding the mode of delivery
35. Undiagnosed breech is associated with increased perinatal mortality and morbidity
36. Up to a third of all breech presentations could first be diagnosed in labour

Vulval cancer and pregnancy

37. Radical surgery for vulval cancer in pregnancy is contraindicated, especially because of the increased risk of abortion from the general anaesthetic
38. Vaginal delivery is contraindicated if vulval cancer is diagnosed in pregnancy

Dyspareunia can be associated with

39. Hydrosalpinx
40. Bechet's syndrome
41. Appendicitis

Delivery in women with cardiac disease

42. Elective forceps delivery is the preferred mode of delivery for woman with cardiac disease
43. Ergometrine should not be used for the routine prophylaxis of post-partum haemorrhage but can be used in the treatment of primary post-partum haemorrhage
44. Syntocinon is the drug of choice for the management of primary post-partum haemorrhage
45. Eight hourly intramuscular injections of ampicillin 500 mg and gentamycin 80 mg provide adequate prophylaxis against endocarditis in labour

Risk factors for developing cervical cancer include

46. Smoking
47. Late menopause
48. Early age of first intercourse
49. Precocious puberty
50. Low social class

Cephalo-pelvic disproportion (CPD)

51. Is associated with a high head at 37 weeks of pregnancy
52. Prolonged latent phase of labour and significant caput are the signs
53. Mild degree of fetal head moulding in labour is a sign of CPD
54. The diagnosis should never be made without trial of labour

Warfarin

55. Is teratogenic when given at 10–12 weeks of pregnancy
56. If a pregnancy occurs whilst a woman is on warfarin termination is advised
57. Microcephaly and optic nerve atrophy are known associations
58. Breastfeeding is contraindicated
59. Based on the INR, therapeutic ranges should always be between 2 and 2.5
60. Warfarin should be converted to heparin therapy late in the third trimester where possible
61. If a woman on warfarin starts to labour 10 mg of vitamin K IM will reverse the hypocoagulation effectively
62. If a woman on warfarin starts to labour Caesarean section is the preferred mode of delivery

With regard to Paget's disease of vulva

63. The incidence of underlying adenocarcinoma is 5%
64. Adenocarcinoma in association with Paget's disease occurs only locally in the lower genital tract
65. If Paget's disease involves the perianal area the risk of rectal cancer is 10%
66. Paget's disease is a squamous intraepithelial neoplasia

Neonatal risks in a diabetic pregnancy are

67. Hyperglycaemia
68. Anaemia
69. Hyperbillirubinaemia
70. Birth trauma
71. Hypermagnesaemia
72. Hypocalcaemia
73. Increased risk of developing diabetes in late life

Problems in the puerperium

74. Eight weeks after delivery about 40% of women still experience at least one health problem
75. The incidence of post-partum anaemia is 25–30%
76. Prophylactic antibiotics at Caesarean section reduce the risk of puerperal febrile morbidity by a third and serious post-partum infection by 25%
77. Perineal pain persists for more than 2 months after delivery in 30% of women
78. Megapulse and ultrasound post-partum significantly improve perineal pain
79. Mefenamic acid is more effective than paracetamol in relieving post-partum perineal pain

The incidence of vulvo-vaginal candidiasis is increased

80. In pregnancy
81. In HIV positive patients
82. In women with oestrogen implants
83. In renal transplant patients
84. By injection of depo-medroxyprogesterone acetate
85. By levonorgestrel implants
86. By use of the modern combined oral contraceptive pill
87. The incidence has increased over the last years

Amniocentesis

88. Prevents polyhydramnios
89. Down's syndrome can be diagnosed by radioimmunoassay of amniotic fluid
90. Positive Kleihauer test is a recognized complication

With regard to the management of recurrent miscarriage

91. Subcutaneous heparin with steroids should be used as a first line therapy for the treatment of recurrent miscarriage associated with abnormal maternal blood clotting
92. GnRH analogues are highly effective in women with high basal LH level
93. HCG luteal phase support is an effective treatment in preventing miscarriage

Fetal hypoxia

94. When acute, leads to loss of fetal breathing movements, flexor tone and heart rate accelerations
95. When chronic manifests with oligohydramnios

In the diagnosis of early pregnancy

96. Radio-immunoassays can detect beta HCG levels of 5 IU/l
97. Radio-immunoassays can detect beta HCG in serum 9 days after ovulation
98. Urinary beta HCG radio-immunoassays become positive before serum ones
99. Transvaginal scans allow for the earlier diagnosis of pregnancy than biochemical methods
100. Transvaginal scans allow for the earlier diagnosis of pregnancy than transabdominal scans
101. A beta HCG level of more than 5 IU/l is diagnostic of pregnancy
102. Doubling serum beta HCG every 4 days is indicative of an intrauterine pregnancy

Perioperative death

103. Is defined as a death under anaesthesia, during surgery and up to 42 days after surgery

Recognized indications for a GTT include

104. Single episode of glycosuria in early pregnancy
105. Family history of diabetes
106. Previous baby more than 4 kg
107. Polyhydramnios
108. Fetal macrosomia
109. When random blood glucose level exceeds 11 mmol/l

Regarding sterilization

110. The incidence of failure of female sterilization is 2–5/1000
111. 80–90% of failures of female sterilization are operator dependent
112. Male sterilization is a safer procedure than female sterilization
113. Laparoscopic sterilization has a higher success rate than sterilization at Caesarean section
114. Quinacrine pellets have been used effectively

The following postoperative complications match

115.	DVT	Day 2–3
116.	Paralytic ileus	Day 7–10
117.	Atelectasis	Day 3–4
118.	Wound dehiscence	Day 3–4
119.	Secondary haemorrhage	Day 3–5

Haemoglobinopathies

120. Alpha-thalassaemia major deteriorates during pregnancy
121. HbH occurs when 2 alpha globin genes are absent, and is associated with severe anaemia
122. Haemoglobin Barts occurs when 3 alpha chain genes are absent
123. Haemoglobin electrophoresis in a patient affected with beta-thalassaemia major shows absence of haemoglobin A_2

Mifepristone

124. Is a better tolerated and more effective post-coital contraceptive agent when compared to the Yuzpe regime
125. Can be used effectively in the conservative treatment of molar pregnancies
126. When given just before the LH surge delays ovulation
127. Has a 3–5 times greater affinity for the progesterone receptor than progesterone itself
128. Has anti-glucocorticoid effects

Match the contraceptives with the correct contraindications

129. OCP   Dubin–Johnson syndrome
130. POP   Recent trophoblastic disease
131. LNG-IUD   Wilson's disease
132. OCP   Vincent's angina

Polyhydramnios

133. Is diagnosed if the liquor volume at term is greater than 1000 ml
134. Is associated with an increased intrauterine pressure in over 60% of cases
135. Is associated with an increased incidence of leg oedema
136. Is associated with poorly controlled diabetes
137. Is found more often with dizygotic than monozygotic twins

Regarding cervical cytological screening

138. The Jordan spatula allows better sampling of the endocervical canal than the Ayres spatula
139. After a cone biopsy a cytobrush is preferred to an Ayres spatula for cytological follow up
140. If the squamo-columnar junction is invisible cytological screening loses its value and should be abandoned
141. Residual VAIN on the vault after hysterectomy can be adequately monitored with vault smears
142. In post-menopausal women an Ayres spatula is the best way to sample the cervix

Drugs contraindicated whilst breastfeeding include

143. Rifampicin
144. Nalidixic acid
145. Fluoxetine
146. Senna

Leukoplakia

147. Is an irregular thickening and whitening of the vulval skin that is seen in several pathological conditions

The following maternal diseases can affect the neonate

148. Idiopathic thombocytopenic purpura
149. Chickenpox
150. Herpes simplex
151. Syphilis
152. Hyperthyroidism

With regard to staging of endometrial cancer

153. Presence of cervical stromal invasion is stage IIb
154. Positive peritoneal cytology is characteristic for stage IIIa
155. A tumour invading bladder and bowel mucosa is stage IVa

The incidence of endometrial cancer

156. It is the third commonest cancer in women in the UK
157. Has been declining over the last decade
158. Is higher in the developing countries

Gonorrhoea

159. Gonococci are Gram-negative diplococci specifically affecting genital tract epithelium
160. Transmission of the organism occurs more readily from women to men than vice versa
161. The gonococcus is fastidious requiring carbon dioxide for its growth
162. Is adequately isolated with a high vaginal swab
163. Is associated with arthritis in 1% of cases
164. Late stage disease may present with collapse from a ruptured aortic aneurysm

Confidential Enquiry into Stillbirths and Deaths in Infancy

165. Sub-optimal care caused 78% of the intrapartum related deaths
166. Is an attempt to identify ways in which late fetal losses, stillbirths and deaths in infancy might be prevented
167. The fourth biannual report was released in 1997
168. Intrapartum mortality rates have decreased steadily over the last years

In hepatitis B infection

169. HBe Ag is a marker of low infectivity
170. HBe Ab is a marker of low infectivity
171. HBc IgG is a medium term marker of previous exposure to HBV
172. HBc IgM is an indicator of acute infection

In the diagnosis of bacterial vaginosis

173. Clue cells are bacterial
174. Vaginal pH is > 3.5
175. A positive amine test is demonstrated by the presence of a fishy smell when adding 10% HCl to a slide containing the vaginal discharge

With regard to urodynamics

176. The normal peak flow rate is at least 15 ml/s for a voided volume of at least 150 ml
177. Reduced maximum urine flow rate (< 15 ml/s) indicates outflow obstruction
178. A low compliant bladder is diagnosed by a detrusor pressure of at least 10 cm H_2O for a filled volume of 500 ml
179. Maximum detrusor pressure during voiding is less than 60 cm H_2O

Miscarriage and termination of pregnancy

180. WHO defines an abortion as the expulsion or extraction from its mother of a fetus or an embryo weighing 500 g or less
181. In UK law spontaneous abortion is defined as pregnancy loss before 24 weeks gestation
182. The upper limit for social termination of pregnancy is 24 weeks

Misoprostol

183. Is prostaglandin E_2
184. Is more expensive than gemeprost
185. Oral administration requires a much higher dose than vaginal administration
186. 800 mg is the minimal effective dose for medical termination of pregnancy

Chorionic villus sampling (CVS)

187. Is safe before 8 weeks, with a fetal loss rate of 3–4%
188. Can be used to diagnose neural tube defects earlier than amniocentesis
189. If the procedure fails, later amniocentesis is contraindicated
190. Sampling is best achieved by taking 10–20 mg of villi from the chorion laeve
191. Results are quicker than amniocentesis and as reliable

Regarding treatment of pruritus vulvae

192. Topical application of oestrogen cream is a universally effective treatment method
193. Topical testosterone cream is an effective therapy
194. Betnovate is a more potent steroid than dermovate

Congenital dislocation of the hip (CDH)

195. Is more common in females than males
196. Is associated with breech presentation at term
197. Is bilateral in more than 50% of cases
198. Is associated with amniocentesis
199. Is associated with polyhydramnios
200. Its incidence is influenced by the method of breech delivery

Radiotherapy

201. Ionizing radiation affects the genetic material of the cell
202. Cells with high mitotic rate are preferentially killed
203. Hypoxic cells have higher radiosensitivity
204. Is a treatment of choice for stage III vaginal cancer
205. Is a first line treatment for recurrent gynaecological cancer
206. Can be used to relieve lymphatic obstruction of the lower limb in advanced gynaecological cancer
207. Is a first line treatment for patients with a locally advanced cancer of the cervix

The following drugs administered during pregnancy are correctly paired

208. L-Thyroxine	Neonatal thyrotoxicosis
209. α-Methyldopa	Fetal tachycardia
210. Chlorothiazide	Maternal pancreatitis
211. Glibenclamide	Neonatal hyperglycaemia
212. Phenytoin sodium	Maternal anaemia secondary to B12 deficiency

Clear cell adenocarcinoma of the vagina

213. Is a childhood tumour of infants who have been exposed to diethylstilboestrol *in utero*
214. Chemotherapy is the treatment of choice

Ergometrine

215. Like oxytocin, causes contraction of the myoepithelial cells in the maternal breasts
216. Its onset of action is 45 seconds after intravenous injection

Bartholin's carcinomas

217. 25% of Bartholin's carcinomas present as an abscess

Rubella is linked to

218. Neonatal anaemia
219. Spontaneous abortion
220. Neonatal purpura
221. Congenital deafness

Surgical management of urinary incontinence

222. Marshall–Marchetti–Kranz procedure is associated with periosteitis pubis in 1%
223. Porcine dermis could be used for Stamey procedure for GSI
224. The needle suspension of the bladder neck is associated with a 15% incidence of voiding difficulties and *de novo* detrusor instability
225. If treatment of urinary incontinence with periurethral injections of collagen fails other surgical procedures are necessary

Extremely premature infants

226. Are at high risk for sudden infant death at home
227. Have a 10% risk of bilateral blindness
228. Have a 1% risk of severe sensorineural deafness
229. Have an almost 1% risk of major sensorineural impairment
230. Are at risk of later hospital admissions for medical and surgical indications

Donor insemination

231. Is no longer required since the introduction of intracytoplasmic sperm injection (ICSI)
232. Decreased success rates occur with frozen as opposed to fresh samples
233. All donors are screened once for HIV
234. Is regulated by HFEA
235. Any donor is limited to the number of families they can create

Meconium aspiration

236. Is always associated with low Apgar score at 5 minutes
237. Is common in post-term pregnancies

Primary amenorrhoea is characteristically associated with

238. Down's syndrome
239. Kallman's syndrome
240. Turner's syndrome
241. Testicular feminization syndrome
242. XXX karyotype
243. Edward's syndrome

Post-coital bleeding can be caused by

244. CIN 3
245. IUCD

Recognized complications of eclampsia include

246. Cerebral haemorrhage
247. Hypothermia
248. Renal cortical necrosis

The following are not associated with an increase in the risk of acquiring PID

249. Early commencement of sexual relations
250. Frequent intercourse
251. Pelvic surgery
252. Recurrent candidal infections
253. IUCD in a stable relationship

Face presentation

254. Incidence is 1 in 200 deliveries
255. First stage is prolonged
256. There is an increased chance of a cord prolapse
257. Presenting diameter is submento-vertical
258. At term mento-posterior position can safely be delivered vaginally
259. Vacuum extraction is safe when performed by a skilled person under epidural analgesia

After the menopause the following may occur

260. Reduction in vaginal acidity
261. Loss of libido
262. Memory loss
263. Gonadotrophin secretion falls
264. Osteoblastic activity increases

The following mortalities match

265. Perinatal   Stillbirths and live births up to 14 days per 1000 live births
266. Post-neonatal   Deaths after 28 days of birth to 1 year
267. Neonatal   Deaths within 7 days of birth

Treatment of the premenstrual syndrome

268. Patient response to placebo is around 90%
269. Pyridoxine and oil of evening primrose are highly effective in treatment of mild cases
270. Levonorgestrel-loaded IUD can be successfully used in conjunction with hormonal therapy in women refusing a hysterectomy
271. Combined surgical and hormonal therapy may be successful in management of severe cases
272. Diuretics have been proven to be effective

Epilepsy in pregnancy

273. Multiple anticonvulsant therapy is preferred as it has a better prophylactic effect in reducing the risk of convulsions
274. Anticonvulsants can be discontinued before pregnancy if a woman has been symptom-free for 2 years
275. A woman on anticonvulsants planning a pregnancy should be started on low dose folate 3 months before discontinuing contraception in order to reduce the risk of neural tube defects
276. Epileptic women in pregnancy should be treated with carbamazepine
277. Anticonvulsants in late pregnancy are known to be associated with Vitamin K deficiency in the neonate
278. Anticonvulsant levels are better monitored in saliva
279. A woman requiring anticonvulsants in pregnancy can be reassured that the fetal abnormalities liable to occur due to these medications can be diagnosed by ultrasound and the pregnancy terminated if necessary
280. Anticonvulsant therapy reduces the risk of intrauterine fetal death
281. The low dose combined oral contraceptive pill is the contraceptive of choice for a woman on anticonvulsants

Post-partum period and diabetes

282. A diabetic woman should be discouraged from breastfeeding
283. The contraceptive of choice is the combined oral contraceptive pill
284. IUCD should not be used

Bacteroides infection is associated with

285. Endotoxic shock
286. Premenarcheal vaginal bleeding
287. Disseminated intravascular coagulation
288. Leucopenia
289. Renal tubular or cortical necrosis
290. Puerperal sepsis
291. *B. fragilis* colonization of the vagina

In pregnancy

292. To reduce the maternal mortality from road traffic accidents, three point harness seat belts are recommended
293. Most drugs are safer for use in the second trimester of pregnancy than in the first, because increasing placental maturation provides more effective protection for the fetus from the effects of therapeutic levels of the drugs
294. Visual display units are associated with increased risk of miscarriage
295. Vertical transmission of hepatitis C is less likely to occur than B, but it can affect the fetus

Match

296. BRAC 1   Chromosome 17
297. Cystic hygroma   Chromosome 21
298. Choroid plexus cysts   Chromosome 18
299. Holoprosencephaly   Chromosome 13

UTIs

300. *E. coli* is cultured in mid-stream urine specimens in 80% of women with urinary tract infection

ANSWERS TO PAPER FIVE

The numbers of the correct answers are given

Norplant
3, 4, 7, 8, 9
Consists of 6 capsules releasing levonorgestrel and is efficacious for 5 years. 24 hours after insertion, the plasma levels are 1–2 ng/ml, falling to 0.25–0.4 ng/ml by 6 months (4–5 times higher initially). From then on they remain constant. If implanted on days 2–5 of the menstrual cycle, barrier methods are advised for 7 days. It can be implemented from 21 days post partum (using a barrier method for 7 days) and on days 1–5 after a termination. Progesterone levels become undetectable within 48 hours of removal of the capsules.

References
L. Mascarenhas, J. Newton. Contraceptive implants. In: Studd J, ed. *Progress in Obstetrics and Gynaecology*, Volume 12. Edinburgh: Churchill Livingstone, 1996.
Long-acting progestogen-only contraception. *Drugs and Therapeutics Bulletin*, 1996; **34**: 93–96.

Currently the 5 year survival for patients with vulval cancer
12 (Vulva)
The survival rate falls from 75% if the lymph nodes are not involved, to 40% in lymph node-positive patients.

Reference
Helm CW, Shingleton HM. The management of squamous cell carcinoma of the vulva. *Current Obstetrics and Gynaecology*, 1992; **2**: 31–37.

Vulval skin
14 (Radiotherapy, Vulva)

Amniotic fluid embolism may present with
15, 16, 17, 18 (Amniotic fluid embolism)
Other presentations include septic or anaphylactic shock, aspiration pneumonitis, pulmonary embolism, myocardial infarction. Disseminated intravascular coagulopathy can lead to haemorrhagic complications.

References
Report on Confidential Enquiries into Maternal Deaths in the United Kingdom, 1991-1993. London: HMSO, 1996.
Still DR. Postpartum haemorrhage and other problems of the third stage. In: James DK, Steer PJ, Weiner CP, Gonik B. eds. *High Risk Pregnancy Management Options*. London: WB Saunders Company, 1994; 1167–1181.

Methotrexate in the treatment of ectopic pregnancy
19, 21   (Ectopic pregnancy)
HCG levels often increase initially, monitoring of serum beta HCG ensures cessation of trophoblastic activity.

Anaemia in pregnancy
24   (Anaemia in pregnancy)
Iron requirements in pregnancy are at their highest level at 32 weeks. Megaloblastic anaemia is commonly due to folate deficiency. Vitamin B12 deficiency is rare.

Reference
Stirrat GM. *Aids to Obstetrics and Gynaecology for MRCOG*, 4th edition. Edinburgh: Churchill Livingstone,1997; 78–79.

VIN
26, 28   (Vulva)
Itching is not necessarily a feature of VIN. The malignant potential of VIN is lower than that of CIN. The risk of progression of VIN to cancer is higher in elderly and immunosuppressed patients.

References
Evans S. Vulval skin disease and the gynaecologist. *British Journal of Hospital Medicine*, 1997; **57**: 579–581.
Maclean AB. Precursors of vulval cancers. *Current Obstetrics and Gynaecology*, 1993; **3**: 149–156
Sarhanis P, Blackett AD, Sharp F. Intraepithelial neoplasia of the anogenital area: a multicentric condition. *Current Obstetrics and Gynaecology*, 1996; **6**: 92–97.

TENS
29, 30   (Analgesia/anaesthesia in labour)

Breech presentation
31, 33, 34, 36   (Breech)
The incidence of breech presentation declines from 16% at 32 weeks to 3–4% at 40 weeks. The incidence of flexed breech is 25%; extended breech is the commonest at 65%. About one third of breeches are first diagnosed in labour, but this is not found to be associated with increased perinatal mortality.

References
Burr RW, Johanson RB. Breech presentation: is external cephalic version worthwhile? *Progress in Obstetrics and Gynaecology*, **12**: 87–96.
Saunders NJ. The management of breech presentation. *British Journal of Hospital Medicine*, 1996; **56**(9): 456–458.

Vulval cancer and pregnancy

(Cancer in pregnancy)

Although surgery does increase the risks of abortion, radical vulvectomy with bilateral groin node dissection may be performed in the first half of pregnancy. Vaginal delivery is not contraindicated either after radical vulvectomy, or in women with the cancer if the lesion is remote from the introitus.

Dyspareunia can be associated with

39, 40, 41   (Dyspareunia)

Delivery in women with cardiac disease

43, 45   (Cardiac disease in pregnancy)

Elective forceps delivery is not necessary in all women with cardiac disease. However, instrumental assistance should be considered if the second stage of labour becomes prolonged or cardiac disease is severe. Ergometrine should not be routinely used for prophylaxis of post-partum haemorrhage, to avoid blood pressure fluctuations, but it is recommended for the management of primary post-partum haemorrhage. Syntocinon is the drug of choice for prophylaxis.

References

De Swiet M, ed. *Medical Disorders in Obstetric Practice*. Oxford: Blackwell Scientific Publications, 1994.

Oakley CM. Pregnancy and heart disease. *British Journal of Hospital Medicine*, 1996; **55**: 423–426.

Risk factors for developing cervical cancer include

46, 48, 50   (Cancer of the cervix)

Precocious puberty is not associated with sexual promiscuity. Late menopause is a risk factor for endometrial and breast cancer.

Cephalopelvic disproportion (CPD)

(Cephalopelvic disproportion)

CPD should be suspected with a high fetal head after 39 weeks of gestation, a prolonged latent phase of labour, poor application of the fetal head to the cervix, when slow progress in labour is associated with contractions becoming irregular and weak, and progressive fetal head moulding. Mild degrees of moulding are not necessarily signs of CPD, as safe delivery of the fetus is possible. Caput is not a sign of CPD, but it may obscure moulding and make the diagnosis of CPD difficult. The diagnosis of CPD can be made without a trial of labour in rare cases like a large hydrocephalus.

Reference

Pelvimetry–Clinical indications. March 1998, Guideline No. 14.

Warfarin

57, 59, 60, 62   (Coagulation and pregnancy)

Warfarin embryopathy is associated with drug administration at 6–9 weeks of pregnancy. Therefore, if the pregnancy has occurred while a woman was on warfarin, termination is not necessary if the drug was discontinued before six weeks' gestation. Warfarin embryopathy also includes chondrodysplasia and neurological abnormalities. Warfarin is not contraindicated in a breastfeeding mother. An INR of 2–2.5 is sufficient for DVT prophylaxis but is too low for treatment of emboli (2–3) or use with prosthetic heart valves (3–4.5). It should be substituted with heparin at 2–3 weeks before delivery in order to reduce the risk of post-partum haemorrhage and fetal intracranial haemorrhage. If a woman on warfarin starts to labour, 10 mg of vitamin K should be administered together with fresh frozen plasma to achieve immediate reversal of anticoagulant effects. Caesarean delivery is preferred to vaginal in order to minimize the risks of fetal intracranial haemorrhage.

Reference

Horn EH. Anticoagulants in pregnancy. *Current Obstetrics and Gynaecology*, 1996; **6**: 111–118.

With regard to Paget's disease of vulva

Paget's disease is a non-squamous, premalignant condition. The incidence of underlying adenocarcinoma is 25%. Adenocarcinoma can occur locally or at distant sites (e.g. breast, urinary tract). When Paget's disease involves the perianal area the risk of rectal carcinoma is 70%.

Reference

MacLean AB. Precursors of vulval cancers. *Current Obstetrics and Gynaecology* 1993; **3**: 149–156.

Neonatal risks in diabetic pregnancy are

69, 70, 72, 73   (Diabetes and pregnancy)

Neonatal risks include hypoglycaemia, polycythaemia, hypomagnesaemia. The risk of developing diabetes in late life is estimated at 1% against 0.1% for the general population.

References

Johnstone FD. Pregnancy management in women with insulin-dependent diabetes. *British Journal of Hospital Medicine*, 1997; **58**(5): 207–210.

Pearson JF. Pregnancy and complicated diabetes. *British Journal of Hospital Medicine*, 1993; **49**(10): 739–742.

Vaughan NJA. Diabetes in pregnancy. *Current Obstetrics and Gynaecology*, 1994; **4**: 155–159.

Problems in the puerperium
75, 79

Puerperal morbidity is extensive. Eight weeks after delivery about 80% of women experience at least one health problem. Prophylactic antibiotics at Caesarean section reduce the risk of puerperal febrile morbidity to a third and serious post-partum infection to a quarter. In 8–10% of women perineal pain persists for more than eight weeks.

Reference
Glazener CMA. Postpartum problems. *British Journal of Hospital Medicine*, 1997; **58**(7): 313–316.

The incidence of vulvo-vaginal candidiasis is increased
80, 81, 82, 83, 87

Progestogen implants and injections reduce the risk of vaginal candida infection. Modern combined oral contraceptive pills do not increase the risk of vulvo-vaginal candidiasis.

References
Emens JM. Intractable vaginal discharge. *Current Obstetrics and Gynaecology*, 1993; **3**: 41–47.
Thomas EJ, Rock J. *Benign Gynaecological Disease*. Oxford: Health Press. 1997; 52–58.

Amniocentesis
90 (Prenatal diagnosis)

Amniocentesis is used to drain amniotic fluid in polyhydramnios in order to provide symptomatic relief to the mother and to prolong pregnancy, but it cannot prevent polyhydramnios. Down's syndrome is diagnosed by chromosomal analysis of the fetal cells in the amniotic fluid.

With regard to the management of recurrent miscarriage
(Abortion spontaneous/recurrent)

Therapy with steroids and heparin has a high incidence of maternal complications and potential side effects on the developing fetus. GnRH analogues are not effective and there is no evidence to support the use of HCG.

Reference
Rai R, Regan L. Recurrent miscarriage. *PACE review* No 96/08.

Fetal hypoxia
94, 95

References
Alfirevic Z, Neilson JP. Fetal growth retardation: methods of detection. *Current Obstetrics and Gynaecology*, 1993; **3**: 190–195.
Harman C, Menticoglou S, Manning F, Albar I, Morrison I. Prenatal fetal monitoring. Abnormalities of fetal behaviour. In: James DK, Steer PJ, Weiner CP, Gonik B (eds). *High Risk Pregnancy Management Options*. London: WB Saunders Company, 1994; 693–734.

In the diagnosis of early pregnancy
96, 97, 100   (Ectopic pregnancy)

Rises in HCG are first seen in serum (9 days after ovulation) then urine (at 13 days). Levels of more than 25 IU/l are necessary to diagnose a pregnancy. Pregnancy is diagnosed earlier with biochemical methods than with transvaginal scans. Ectopic pregnancy is more likely under the circumstances described in 102.

Perioperative death
(Report on the National Confidential Enquiry into Perioperative Deaths)

Is defined as a death under anaesthesia, during surgery and up to 30 days after surgery.

Recognized indications of GTT include
105, 107, 108   (Diabetes and pregnancy)

GTT is indicated in the presence of a single episode of glycosuria in late pregnancy or two episodes in early pregnancy and when the previous baby was more than 4.5 kg at birth. Random blood glucose more than 11 mmol/l indicates that glucose tolerance is abnormal, therefore a GTT is not necessary.

Reference

Maresh MJA. Glucose intolerance in pregnancy. *PACE review* No 97/03.

Regarding sterilization
110, 112, 113, 114   (Contraception and sterilization)

30–40% of failures are thought to be operator-dependent.

Reference

Sokal DC, Zipper J, King T. Transcervical quinacrine sterilisation: clinical experience. In: Wilson (ed). The development of new technologies for female sterilisation. *Intern Journal of Gynecology and Obstetrics,* 1995; **51** (suppl. 1): 557–569.

The following postoperative complications match
115, 118   (Perioperative complications)

Paralytic ileus is normally present by days 3–4. Atelectasis occurs in the first couple of days. Wound dehiscence can occur at any time. Secondary haemorrhage by definition occurs after 7 days.

Haemoglobinopathies

Alpha thalassaemia major is incompatible with life; all four genes for alpha globin are absent and haemoglobin electrophoresis shows gamma tetramers known as haemoglobin Barts which is unable to carry oxygen. Absence of three genes of alpha globin leads to beta tetramer formation known as haemoglobin H, and increased concentrations of fetal haemoglobin. In beta-thalassaemia major, HbA_2 and HbF are present and HbA_1 is absent.

Reference

Malpas JS, Story P. Diseases of the blood. In: Kumar PJ, Clark ML, eds. *Clinical Medicine.* London: Ballière Tindall, 1988; 260–301.

Mifepristone
124, 127, 128
When given just before the LH surge, mifepristone has no effect on ovulation or the length of the luteal phase. Mifepristone is useful in the conservative management of miscarriage.

Match the contraceptives with the correct contraindications
129, 130
Copper IUCDs are contraindicated in Wilson's disease. Vincent's angina is a pharyngeal infection treated with metronidazole.

Polyhydramnios
135, 136   (Polyhydramnios/oligohydramnios)
Polyhydramnios at term is diagnosed when the liquor volume is greater than 2000 ml, the amniotic fluid index is greater than 20 or the largest amniotic pool is greater than 8 cm. It is more common in monozygotic twins. In poorly controlled diabetes, fetal hyperglycaemia and polyuria are the possible causes. Polyhydramnios causes uterine over-distension and pressure on the inferior vena cava, thus reducing venous return from the lower limbs which causes oedema.

Reference
Stark C. Disorders of the amniotic fluid. In: Frederickson HL, Wilkins-Haug L, eds. *Ob/Gyn Secrets*. Philadelphia: Hanley & Belfus Inc., 1991; 217–220.

Regarding cervical cytological screening
138, 139   (Premalignant disease of the cervix)
Amongst the currently available sampling devices, the one mainly used for sampling the ectocervix is the Ayres spatula. The endocervix is better sampled with Jordan and Aylesbury spatulas, cytobrush and Cervex. These devices should be used for cytological follow-up after cone biopsy and when the squamo-columnar junction is invisible (e.g. in post-menopausal women). In practical terms the cytobrush allows better sampling of the endocervical canal than Ayres spatula but should not be used alone. Cytological screening is necessary even if the squamo-columnar junction is invisible, but the endocervical canal should be sampled. Residual VAIN may remain beyond suture lines and be inaccessible to cytological follow-up.

References
Macgregor JE. What constitutes an adequate cervical smear? *British Journal of Obstetrics and Gynaecology*, 1991; **98**: 6–7.
Sasieni P. Cervical sampling devices. *BMJ* 1996; **313**: 1275–1276.

Drugs contraindicated whilst breastfeeding include
145, 146
Rifampicin is excreted in the breast milk in amounts too small to be harmful. Nalidixic acid is thought to be safe but one case of haemolytic anaemia has been reported. Fluoxetine is not recommended. Senna and other anthraquinones increase gastric motility and may cause diarrhoea.

Reference
British National Formulary. **36**; March 1998.

Leukoplakia
147

Reference
Maclean AB. Precursors of vulval cancers. *Current Obstetrics and Gynaecology*, 1993;
3: 149–156.

The following maternal diseases can affect the neonate
148, 149, 150, 151, 152   (Infection in pregnancy, Thyroid and pregnancy)

Reference
MacLean AB, Cockburn F. Maternal and perinatal infection. In: Whitfield CR, ed.
Dewhurst's Textbook of Obstetrics and Gynaecology for Postgraduates, 5th edn.
Oxford: Blackwell Science, 1995; 477–491.

With regard to staging of endometrial cancer
153, 154, 155

References
Irwin CJR. The Management of endometrial carcinoma. *British Journal of Hospital
Medicine*, 1996; **55**: 308–309.
Semple D. Endometrial cancer. *British Journal of Hospital Medicine*, 1997; **57**: 260–262.

The incidence of endometrial cancer
This is the ninth commonest cancer in women in the UK. Its incidence is higher in
developed countries and is on the increase.

References
Rose P. Endometrial carcinoma. *The New England Journal of Medicine*, 1996; **335**: 640–
648.
Semple D. Endometrial cancer. *British Journal of Hospital Medicine*, 1997; **57**: 260–
262.

Gonorrhoea
161, 163   (Sexually transmitted disease)
Gonococci are Gram-negative diplococci that attack the columnar epithelium of the
endocervix and the transitional epithelium of the urethra. Transmission of the
organism occurs more readily from infected men to women than vice versa (50%
compared with 20%). It is not adequately isolated with a high vaginal swab. Late stage
syphilitic disease may present with collapse from a ruptured aortic aneurysm.

Confidential Enquiry into Stillbirths and Deaths in Infancy

166 (Confidential Enquiry into Stillbirths and Deaths in Infancy (CESDI))

The Confidential Enquiry into Stillbirths and Deaths in Infancy was established in 1992. The reports are released annually; the fourth report was released in 1997. The intrapartum mortality rates have stayed constant. However, 78% of the deaths were criticized for sub-optimal care that would have made a difference to 52% of the outcomes and may have made a difference to a further 25% of outcomes.

In hepatitis B infection

170, 172

HBe Ag is a marker of high infectivity. HBc IgG is a permanent marker of previous exposure to HBV.

Reference

Stabile I, Chard T, Grudzinskas G. *Clinical Obstetrics and Gynaecology*. New York: Springer-Verlag, 1996; 190.

In the diagnosis of bacterial vaginosis

Clue cells are large epithelial cells with bacteria attached to their surface. Vaginal pH is > 4.5. 10% KOH is used for the amine test.

References

Lamont RF. Bacterial vaginosis. *The Year Book of the RCOG* 1994; 149–158.

MacDermott RIJ. Bacterial vaginosis. *British Journal of Obstetrics and Gynaecology*, 1995; **102**: 92–94.

With regard to urodynamics

176, 179 (Urinary incontinence: urodynamics)

Urine flow less than 15 ml/s may also indicate inadequate detrusor function. Low compliance is diagnosed by a detrusor pressure of at least 10 cm H_2O for a filled volume of 300 ml, or a rise of at least 15 cm H_2O for a filled volume of 500 ml.

References

Cardozo L, Hill S. Urinary incontinence. RCOG PACE review 96/09.

Jarvis GJ. Female urinary incontinence – which patients? – which tests? *The Year Book of The RCOG* 1994; 111–120.

Richmond D. The incontinent woman: 1. *British Journal of Hospital Medicine*, 1993; **50**: 418–423.

Miscarriage and termination of pregnancy

180, 181 (Therapeutic abortion)

There is no such thing as a social termination.

Misoprostol

(Therapeutic abortion)

This is a PGE$_1$ analogue, which is becoming increasingly popular due to its lower cost. Similar doses are used for vaginal and oral administration. Although it has been used in a dose of 800 mg there is a strong evidence that 200 mg is as effective.

Reference

Henshaw RC, Templeton AA. Methods used in first trimester abortion. *Current Obstetrics and Gynaecology*, 1993; **3**: 11–16.

Chorionic villus sampling (CVS)

(Prenatal diagnosis)

CVS is usually performed between 10 and 14 weeks with a 3–4% rate of fetal loss occuring within 6 weeks. It cannot diagnose neural tube defects, but is indicated for parental chromosomal abnormalities, X-linked diseases and for certain metabolic disorders (e.g. Hurler's syndrome). Amniocentesis is recommended if CVS fails. Cells are collected from the chorion frondosum, and 10–50 mg of tissue is normally required. Chromosomal analysis is performed by cell culture (within 10 days), rapid karyotyping or fluorescent *in situ* hybridization (FISH, within 2 days). The false positive rate is more than for amniocentesis.

References

Holzgrave W, Miny P. Chorionic villus sampling. In: James DK, Steer PJ, Weiner CP, Gonik B, eds. *High Risk Pregnancy Management Options*. London: WB Saunders Company, 1994; 635–642.

Neilson JP. Antenatal diagnosis of fetal abnormality. In: Whitfield CR ed. *Dewhurst's Textbook of Obstetrics and Gynaecology for Postgraduates*, 5th edn. Oxford: Blackwell Science, 1995; 221–239.

Regarding treatment of pruritus vulvae

(Pruritus vulvae)

Oestrogen and testosterone creams may relieve vulval itching in a proportion of cases, but these are not effective treatments. Topical graduated steroids are the most effective treatment and are widely used as a first line therapy. The potency of steroids decreases in the following order: dermovate (clobetasol), betnovate (betamethasone), hydrocortisone.

References

Evans S. Vulval skin disease and the gynaecologist. *British Journal of Hospital Medicine*, 1997; **57**: 579–581.

Maclean AB. Precursors of vulval cancers. *Current Obstetrics and Gynaecology*, 1993; **3**: 149–156.

Congenital dislocation of the hip (CDH)
195, 196, 198

The incidence of CDH is 15.7/1000 Caucasians, and 4.9/1000 Afro-Caribbeans. The incidence is 4–6 times higher in girls than boys. There is a higher incidence in breech babies (15.7% compared to 3% for the general population). It is bilateral in 10–15% of cases, 60% are left sided, and 20% right sided. It is associated with oligohydramnios that can occur secondary to amniocentesis. Its incidence is not influenced by the method of breech delivery.

Radiotherapy
201, 202, 204, 206, 207   (Radiotherapy)

Ionizing radiation causes cellular death by interfering with its genetic material. Hypoxic cells are more radio-resistant than normally oxygenated ones. Whether or not radiotherapy should be used as a first line treatment for recurrent gynaecological cancer depends on primary treatment given, site of recurrence, patient's condition and other factors.

The following drugs administered during pregnancy are correctly paired
210

Thyroxine does not pass through the placenta in significant amounts, it may interfere with neonatal screening but does not cause thyrotoxicosis. Methyldopa causes a fetal bradycardia. Glibenclamide causes neonatal hypoglycaemia. Phenytoin sodium causes megaloblastic anaemia due to folic acid deficiency (prophylactic folic acid should be taken by pregnant women on phenytoin).

Reference
British National Formulary. **36**; March 1998.

Clear cell adenocarcinoma of the vagina
(Vaginal tumours)
This commonly occurs in young women (aged 15–27), not infants. Radiotherapy or radical surgery are used for treatment.

Ergometrine
216

Ergometrine does not act on the myoepithelial cells of the breasts. It produces tonic contraction of the uterus with superimposed rapid clonic contractions. It also causes vasoconstriction (contraindicated in peripheral vascular and heart disease). Unlike oxytocin, it has no antidiuretic effect.

Reference
Beazley JM. Natural labour and its active management. In: Whitfield CR, ed.
   Dewhurst's Textbook of Obstetrics and Gynaecology for Postgraduates, 5th edn, Oxford: Blackwell Science, 1995; 293–311.

Bartholin's carcinomas
217

Reference
Maclean AB. Precursors of vulval cancers. *Current Obstetrics and Gynaecology*, 1993; **3**: 149–156.

Rubella is linked to
218, 219, 220, 221   (Infection in pregnancy)
Other effects on the baby are splenomegaly, jaundice, meningoencephalitis, thrombocytopenia, cataract, glaucoma, heart disease, microcephaly, mental retardation. Late findings are diabetes, thyroid problems, precocious puberty and progressive rubella panencephalitis.

References
MacLean AB, Cockburn F. Maternal and perinatal infection. In: Whitfield CR, ed. *Dewhurst's Textbook of Obstetrics and Gynaecology for Postgraduates*, 5th edn. Oxford: Blackwell Science, 1995; 477–493.
Pastorek JG. Viral diseases. In: James DK, Steer PJ, Weiner CP, Gonik B, eds. *High Risk Pregnancy Management Options*. London: WB Saunders Company, 1994; 481–507.

Surgical management of urinary incontinence
222   (Urinary incontinence: urodynamics)
The needle suspension of the bladder neck is associated with an incidence of 5% of voiding difficulties and 5% of *de novo* detrusor instability. Porcine dermis is used for sling procedures. If initial treatment of urinary incontinence with periurethral injections of collagen fails a repeat injection may be successful and should be considered.

References
Cardozo L, Hill S. Urinary incontinence. RCOG PACE review 96/09.
Eckford SD, Keane D. Surgical treatment of urinary stress incontinence. *British Journal of Hospital Medicine*, 1992; **48**: 308–313.
Hilton P. The Stamey procedure for stress incontinence. *Current Obstetrics and Gynaecology*, 1991; **1**: 103–108.
Richmond D. The incontinent woman: 1. *British Journal of Hospital Medicine*, 1993; **50**: 418–423.

Extremely premature infants
226, 227, 230
About 33% of them require later hospital admissions. The risk of severe sensorineural deafness is 10%.

Reference
Knoches Al, Doyle LW. Long-term outcome of infants born preterm. In: Rice GE, Brennecke SP, eds. *Ballière's Clinical Obstetrics and Gynaecology International Practice and Research. Preterm Labour and Delivery*. London: Ballière Tindall, 1993; 633–651.

Donor insemination

232, 234, 235 (Infertility – II)

Despite the introduction of intra-cytoplasmic sperm injection (ICSI) it is still required. All donors are screened twice for HIV.

Meconium aspiration

237

It is not always associated with low Apgar score at 5 minutes.

Reference

Cockburn F. Neonatal care for obstetricians. In: Whitfield CR, ed. *Dewhurst's Textbook of Obstetrics and Gynaecology for Postgraduates*, 5th edn. Oxford: Blackwell Science, 1995; 454–476.

Primary amenorrhoea is characteristically associated with

239, 240, 241

XXX karyotype is associated with premature menopause. There is no association with Down's syndrome, and Edward's syndrome is fatal.

Post-coital bleeding is caused by

(Intermenstrual, post-coital and post-menopausal bleeding)

CIN 3 is preclinical and asymptomatic. IUCD is not a recognized cause of post-coital bleeding.

Recognized complications of eclampsia include

246, 248 (Pre-eclampsia, eclampsia and phaeochromocytoma)

Others are placental abruption, hypovolaemia, thrombocytopenia, pulmonary oedema, ARDS, heart failure, renal failure, hepatic failure, DIC, hyperpyrexia etc.

Reference

Redman C. Hypertension in pregnancy. In: De Swiet M, ed. *Medical Disorders in Obstetrics Practice*, 2nd edn. Oxford: Blackwell Science, 1990; 249–305.

The following are not associated with an increase in the risk of acquiring PID

250, 252, 253 (Pelvic inflammatory disease)

Most of the answers are associated with an increased risk of PID, as are recurrent chlamydial infections and multiple sexual partners. In contrast to *Key Topics in Obstetrics and Gynaecology*, current evidence suggests that there is no increased risk with modern coils used in monogamous relationships. Highest infection rates are seen following insertion through the first 20 days in high risk women.

Reference

Bevan C. Pelvic inflammatory disease. RCOG PACE review 98/04.

Face presentation
254, 255, 256, 257   (Presentations and positions)
In mento-posterior position the presenting diameter is mento-vertical (13 cm in a term fetus) and cannot safely be delivered vaginally. Vacuum extraction is absolutely contraindicated.

Reference
Ritchie JWK. Malpositions of the occiput and malpresentations. In: Whitfield CR, ed. *Dewhurst's Textbook of Obstetrics and Gynaecology for Postgraduates*, 5th edn. Oxford: Blackwell Science, 1995; 346–367.

After the menopause the following occur
260, 261, 262   (Menopause)
Gonadotrophin secretion increases. Osteoblasts are bone-forming, their activity is reduced.

The following mortalities match
266   (Perinatal mortality)
Perinatal mortality is stillbirths and live-births up to seven days per 1000 total (still and live) births. Deaths within 28 days of birth describes neonatal mortality.

Treatment of premenstrual syndrome
268, 270, 271   (Premenstrual syndrome)
Although pyridoxine and oil of evening primrose are widely used, there is no evidence to prove their efficacy. Neither is there any evidence to support benefits from the use of diuretics.

Reference
O'Brian PMS, Abukhalil IEH, Henshaw C. *Current Obstetrics and Gynaecology*, 1995; **5**: 30–35.

Epilepsy in pregnancy
274, 277, 278, 279, 280   (Epilepsy and pregnancy)
The management of pregnancy in an epileptic patient should be planned at a preconception clinic, where anticonvulsants can be discontinued if the woman has remained free of fits for 2 years, or multiple therapy changed to mono-therapy as this reduces the risk of occurrence of fetal anomalies. High dose folate supplements should be given to a woman on anticonvulsants preconceptually. There is no need to change other anticonvulsants to carbamazepine if the symptoms are well controlled as the risks of each are similar and a change of drug could increase the risk of convulsions. Anticonvulsants reduce the risk of intrauterine fetal death, but increase the risk of vitamin K deficiency and, subsequently, bleeding in the neonatal period. Anticonvulsants increase the risk of failure of low dose combined oral contraceptives, therefore high dose pills should be prescribed.

References
Rubin PC. Epilepsy in pregnancy. *Current Obstetrics and Gynaecology*, 1992; **2**: 149–152.
Rutherford JM, Rubin PC. Management of epilepsy in pregnancy: therapeutic aspects. *British Journal of Hospital Medicine*, 1996; **55**: 620–622.

Post-partum period and diabetes
Breastfeeding and the use of an IUCD are not contraindicated. Among hormonal methods of contraception the POP or a triphasic pill are advised.

References
Johnstone FD. Pregnancy management in women with insulin-dependent diabetes. *British Journal of Hospital Medicine*, 1997; **58**(5): 207–210.
Vaughan NJA. Diabetes in pregnancy. *Current Obstetrics and Gynaecology*, 1994; **4**: 155–159.

Bacteroides infection is associated with
285, 287, 288, 290
Pre-mencheal vaginal bleeding refers to sarcoma botryoides. Bacteroids infection is also associated with pelvic and septic thrombophlebitis. *B. fragilis* is uncommon in the vagina, the main species are the melaninogenicus/oralis group.

In pregnancy
292, 295
Most drugs are safer for use in the second trimester of pregnancy than in the first, because organogenesis is complete. Visual display units are not hazardous.

References
Sen A. Seat belts in pregnancy. *BMJ*, 1992; **304**: 586–587.
Working with visual display units in pregnancy. RCOG Guideline 6, 1996.

Match
296, 297, 298, 299
Down's syndrome (chromosome 21) is associated with cystic hygroma. Choroid plexus cysts are associated with Edward's syndrome (chromosome 18) and Patau's syndrome (chromosome 13) is associated with holoprosencephaly.

UTIs
300

PAPER SIX

Allow 2 hours for completion of this paper

Recognized causes of vaginal bleeding in an 8-year-old girl include

1. Sarcoma botryoides
2. Polyostotic fibrous dysplasia
3. Craniopharyngioma
4. Use of diethylstilboestrol by her mother in a previous pregnancy
5. Vaginal adenosis
6. Trichomonas vaginalis infection
7. Dysgerminoma of the ovary
8. Post-encephalitic syndrome
9. Wilson's disease
10. Foreign body

Match

11. Endometrial cancer   Five year survival 45%
12. Vulval cancer   Peak incidence in 60s age group
13. Endometrial cancer   Peak incidence in 50s age group
14. Cervical intraepithelial neoplasia   Peak incidence in 20s age group

Blood transfusion in pregnancy

15. Suppresses the haemopoiesis in women with sickle cell disease
16. May precipitate sickle cell crisis
17. The CLASP trial reliably proved that low dose aspirin is associated with an increased risk of transfusion

Non-surgical management of urinary incontinence

18. Pelvic floor exercises are more successful in older patients than in younger ones
19. Faradism with pelvic floor exercises confers significantly higher success than pelvic floor exercises alone
20. The success rate of vaginal cones in the treatment of GSI is 70%
21. Bladder drill has up to 90% success and a low recurrence rate

Litigation

22. Currently obstetric claims constitute more than 30% of claims against trusts

Preterm breech

23. Has a higher incidence of growth retardation than its cephalic counterpart
24. Has a higher incidence of stillbirth and neonatal death rate than its cephalic counterpart regardless of the mode of delivery
25. Vaginal delivery is associated with a higher risk of entrapment of the after-coming head than a breech at term
26. During labour the risk of cord prolapse is higher compared with a term breech
27. Prophylactic forceps delivery of after-coming head reduces neonatal morbidity
28. At less than 28 weeks breeches should preferably be delivered via Caesarean section to reduce trauma to the baby

The effect of pregnancy on cancer

29. The prognosis of cervical cancer is not altered stage for stage by pregnancy
30. The prognosis of vulval carcinoma is not altered stage for stage
31. The prognosis of breast cancer is unchanged compared with non-pregnant women
32. There is no adverse effect on the prognosis of melanoma
33. The 5 year survival of women who had breast cancer diagnosed in pregnancy is 25%

Regarding third generation combined oral contraceptive pills

34. The risk of venous thrombo-embolism in desogestrel/gestodene pill users is equal to that in pregnancy
35. Desogestrel/gestodene-containing pills are more lipid friendly than the second generation progestogen-containing pills
36. Desogestrel/gestodene-containing pills could be advantageous in older smokers requesting the pill, or unsuitable for other forms of contraception
37. Current UK recommendations for oral contraception users include the following: 'Second generation pills should not be changed to third generation ones under any circumstances'

Perinatal mortality

38. The perinatal mortality rate (PMR) in the UK in the mid 1990s was 7–8 per 10 000 total births
39. Is lowest for the second baby and doubles for the first and fourth child
40. Is increased six-fold in multiple births
41. Is lowest in the social classes two and three
42. Increases steadily from teenage until the mid-thirties when its rate rapidly rises
43. PMR is a sensitive indicator of the standard of obstetric care

Hyperplasia

44. Adenomatous hyperplasia is synonymous with simple hyperplasia
45. Simple hyperplasia is characterized by increased glandular-stromal ratio in the absence of cellular atypia
46. Simple hyperplasia has no malignant potential
47. Complex and adenomatous hyperplasia have identical malignant potential

Post-partum haemorrhage

48. Routine oxytocins in the third stage reduces post-partum blood loss by 30–40%
49. The blood flow through the placenta at term is 500–800 ml/min
50. Syntometrine is as effective as oxytocin alone in hypertensive women

The risks associated with diabetes in pregnancy

51. The incidence of major fetal abnormalities in diabetic women is 3 times greater than in non-diabetic women
52. There is an increased risk of urinary tract infection
53. The prevalence of pre-eclampsia in diabetic pregnant women is 30–40%
54. The prevalence of preterm labour in diabetic women is 5%
55. Diabetic ketoacidosis in pregnancy is associated with fetal loss of 50%

Regarding post-coital contraception

56. Because it contains progesterone the levonorgestrel-releasing coil should be used preferentially as a post-coital device
57. A single dose of 600 mg of mifepristone taken within 72 hours of unprotected intercourse is an effective post-coital contraceptive agent
58. Levonorgestrel 0.75 mg (two doses 12 hours apart) started within 72 hours of unprotected intercourse is effective for the prevention of unwanted pregnancy

The following are associated with endometrial cancer

59. Granulosa cell tumours of the ovary
60. Tamoxifen
61. Polycystic ovarian syndrome
62. Diabetes (insulin resistance)
63. Opposed oestrogen

Caesarean delivery

64. Lower segment sections are associated with less blood loss than classical ones and a 20 times lower risk of scar dehiscence
65. Vaginal delivery after two previous sections is not allowed
66. A Pfannenstiel incision from a previous Caesarean section implies a transverse lower uterine incision
67. If the lower segment incision is insufficient for delivery of the fetus, a 'J' extension is recommended as opposed to an inverted 'T'

Vesico-vaginal fistula may be caused by

68. Radiotherapy
69. Malignancy
70. Childbirth

Fetal effect of analgesia in labour

71. Both regional analgesia and opioids are associated with abnormal CTGs
72. Naloxone injection should routinely be administered to neonates if opioids have been used in labour
73. Neonates require more naloxone if the woman has been using patient-controlled analgesia

Hydatidiform mole may present with

74. Hypertension
75. Fitting
76. Wernicke's encephalopathy

Risk of thrombo-embolic disease and pregnancy

77. Risk is twice as high as in the non-pregnant state
78. Prolonged bed rest is associated with an increased risk
79. Multiple pregnancy is a risk factor
80. Prolonged rupture of membranes is associated with an increased risk
81. Cardiac disease and acute chest infection are risk factors
82. The risk of thrombo-embolic complications is higher with an emergency Caesarean section than with an elective
83. The risk of recurrence after one previous episode and without prophylaxis is 1–5%
84. The measurement of arterial blood gases is a highly sensitive method for diagnosing pulmonary embolism

Delayed puberty

85. Associated with Kallman's syndrome
86. Associated with juvenile hypothyroidism
87. Associated with hypoprolactinaemia
88. Anorexia nervosa is a common cause
89. GnRH analogues can be used for treatment
90. A combined low dose pill is the best treatment
91. Is defined as the absence of pubic and axillary hair by the age of 14 years

Endometriosis

92. The commonest symptoms associated with mild endometriosis are spasmodic dysmenorrhoea, deep dyspareunia and pelvic pain
93. Viable endometrial cells found in peritoneal fluid at the time of menstruation confirm that retrograde menstruation is the cause
94. GnRH analogues combined with HRT can be commenced together when diagnosis is confirmed
95. Endometriotic deposits contain lower concentrations of progestin receptors than normal endometrium
96. Is associated with an increased risk of spontaneous abortion
97. If a woman is found to have endometriosis affecting her Fallopian tubes, they should be removed prior to IVF to improve the success rate

Match the drugs to the correct side effects when used in late pregnancy

98. Chlormethiazole   Respiratory depression
99. Hydralazine   Bradycardia
100. Phenytoin   Congenital abnormalities
101. Diazepam   Hypotonia in the neonate

With regard to ovarian cancer

102. Over 75% of women with ovarian cancer will die from the disease
103. 50% will present with stage three to four disease

Hyperprolactinaemia can be caused by

104. Chronic renal failure
105. Primary hypothyroidism
106. Cimetidine
107. Quinagolide
108. Chest wall injury

Maternal mortality

109. Includes those caused by ectopic pregnancy
110. Is highest in social classes four and five
111. Avoidable factors are present in 35–40% of cases
112. Hypertension is the biggest single cause
113. Is higher in patients over the age of 40 years

Treatment of CIN

114. Amongst excisional biopsy methods, the large loop excision of the transformation zone (LLETZ) is the most traumatic
115. Untreated CIN 1 will regress over 2 years in almost 50% of women
116. Almost 20% of women with untreated CIN 3 will have invasive lesions after 10 years
117. Local ablation is the most acceptable method of treating dyskaryotic cells
118. Laser cone biopsy is preferential to loop diathermy or knife cone biopsies because it provides a better quality specimen for histological diagnosis
119. Clear excisional margins on a cone biopsy indicate complete excision of cervical glandular intraepithelial neoplasia (CGIN)
120. CO_2 laser causes significantly deeper destruction of tissue than cold coagulation
121. The depth of tissue destruction with cryocautery is 4 mm
122. Cryocautery is the treatment of choice when gland clefts are affected by CIN
123. Electro-diathermy causes better local destruction than cryocautery

Detrusor instability

124. When detrusor instability coexists with GSI the detrusor problem should always be treated first

Vulval carcinoma is associated with

125. Smoking
126. Syphilis
127. Lymphogranuloma venereum
128. Nulliparity

Interactions of the combined oral contraceptive pill with other drugs

129. Carbamazepine reduces its efficacy
130. A woman taking a drug that is a liver enzyme inducer who wants to take the pill can safely be prescribed a high dose preparation
131. Penicillin reduces its efficacy

Twin pregnancy

132. The incidence increases with parity
133. The perinatal mortality of the first twin is higher
134. Pre-eclampsia is more common
135. The incidence is about 1 per 80–90 births
136. Is generally caused by superfecundation
137. Preterm delivery occurs in about 50% of cases
138. The leading twin presents by the head in about 75% of cases
139. Dichorionic twin is synonymous with dizygosity

Management of endometrial cancer

140. When presented with intermenstrual bleeding, a pipelle biopsy and transvaginal scan (to measure endometrial thickness) should be used for diagnosis
141. The advantage of a pipelle biopsy is a fast diagnosis when compared with formal D&C
142. Endometrial resection could be employed in early endometrial cancer if fertility is to be retained
143. Stage 1 is better managed by radical hysterectomy
144. Responds well to progestogen therapy only if the tumour is of high grade
145. High dose progesterones could be used in stage 4 disease
146. Tamoxifen decreases the number of progesterone receptors in the endometrium
147. Both radical surgery and chemotherapy are recognized modalities of treatment for recurrent disease
148. Extra-pelvic disease is better treated surgically

Uterine sarcomas

149. Overall survival rate is 30%

Recognized associations of persistent ductus arteriosus in the neonate include

150. True congenital rubella syndrome
151. Marfan's syndrome
152. A continuous murmur over the left upper chest
153. Pulmonary oligaemia
154. The administration of indomethacin prenatally

Radiotherapy in the management of gynaecological cancer

155. Has a success rate similar to surgery
156. Is associated with a lower complication rate than surgery
157. Adjuvant radiotherapy is advised when cervical cancer is incompletely excised or when nodal metastases are present
158. Radiotherapy is a preferred modality of non-surgical treatment of ovarian cancer
159. Central pelvic recurrence of cervical cancer is better treated with radiotherapy
160. Brachytherapy is a type of radiotherapy with the use of an external source of irradiation

Viral infections of the genital tract

161. HPV types 6 and 11 are associated with benign epithelial lesions
162. Genital warts may regress spontaneously
163. Podophyllin is safe in pregnancy
164. Trichloroacetic acid is contraindicated during pregnancy
165. Primary genital HSV infection necessitates screening for other STDs and contact tracing
166. Genital herpes infection is caused solely by HSV type 2

Lymphogranuloma venereum

167. Is caused by chlamydia trachomatis
168. When primary, commonly heals rapidly without leaving a scar
169. May lead to vaginal, urethral and anal stricture formation
170. Clindamycin is the antibiotic of choice

Predisposing factors for an ectopic pregnancy include

171. Previous candidal infection
172. Congenital anomalies of the genital tract
173. The progesterone only pill
174. Combined oral contraceptive pill
175. Treatment with diethylstilboestrol in a previous pregnancy
176. Artificial insemination
177. Late reproductive life

The following match

178. Commonest cause of abnormal vaginal discharge   Trichomonas vaginalis
179. Greenish vaginal discharge   Bacterial vaginosis
180. Greyish vaginal discharge   Trichomonas infection
181. Adherent creamy-white vaginal discharge   Chlamydial infection

Vaginal adenosis

182. Is a benign condition occurring due to exposure to diethylstilboestrol *in utero*

Genuine stress incontinence (GSI)

183. Accounts for 60% of cases of urinary incontinence
184. Topical oestrogen application is an effective therapy for GSI occurring in a young healthy woman

Perinatal medicine

185. A neonate with a birth weight of < 1500 g is termed extremely low birth weight
186. The majority of stillbirths are of unknown cause and remain unpredictable and unpreventable
187. Early fetal loss is defined as loss between 20 and 23 weeks and 6 days of pregnancy

Mifepristone

188. Has a glucocorticoid action
189. Has uterotonic action
190. Is luteolytic
191. Should be avoided in women with recent topical steroid therapy
192. Is contraindicated in chronic renal failure
193. Should not be used in patients with haemorrhagic disorders

Medical termination of pregnancy is associated with

194. 5% ongoing pregnancy
195. Lower incidence of PID than surgical termination

Pre-eclampsia

196. Is usually diagnosed at about 18 weeks' gestation
197. Is associated with thrombocytopenia
198. Should never be treated with diazepam
199. Cannot be diagnosed in the absence of albuminuria
200. May cause haemolysis

Klinefelter's syndrome is associated with

201. Azoospermia
202. Dextrocardia

Predisposing factors for ARDS are

203. Dorsal kyphoscoliosis
204. Epidural analgesia

The management of a woman in pregnancy with a history of herpes infection (but with no visible lesions at present) includes

205. Weekly antenatal cultures from the genital tract
206. Anticipated vaginal delivery
207. Obtaining cultures from the mother and the neonate following delivery
208. Isolation and notification
209. Risk of neonatal infection is approximately 1 in 10 and can be reduced by acyclovir or vibramycin.

Spermicides

210. Are bacteriostatic
211. Nonoxynol 9 has a detergent as its active agent
212. Nonoxynol 9 is known to cause vaginal ulcerations

Regarding HIV infection the following are true

213. IV drug abuse accounts for the infection of 10–15% of pregnant patients in the UK
214. Pregnancy may precipitate AIDS in HIV-positive women
215. Postnatally it may be transmitted to the baby in more than 60% cases
216. Kaposi's sarcoma is a common presentation
217. Of the 250 or more HIV births per year, 80% are undiagnosed at the time of birth
218. 50% of cases infected with HIV will be asymptomatic for up to 4 years
219. HIV may be transmitted via artificial insemination of donor sperm
220. Spread of HIV is 20–50 times less likely via vaginal intercourse than via anal intercourse and can be reduced by using Nonoxynol

Preterm labour

221. Is associated with a past history of preterm labour
222. Is associated with uterine abnormalities, smoking and a maternal pre-pregnancy weight of less than 50 kg
223. The use of ritodrine has been shown to improve perinatal outcome
224. A high vaginal swab should be taken in the presence of ruptured membranes
225. Epidural analgesia should not be used because of the possibility of an occult placental abruption

The expulsion rate of IUCD is higher

226. In younger women
227. In fundal-seeking devices
228. If inserted straight after first trimester termination of pregnancy

Regarding postoperative complications

229. Hernia after a Pfannenstiel incision is commoner at the wound angles
230. Lymph collection after pelvic surgery occurs only in the form of leg swelling

Recurrent miscarriage

231. Paternal chromosomal abnormalities are found in a third of couples
232. Robertsonian translocation is the commonest chromosomal abnormality found in the parents
233. The incidence of PCOS is higher in these women compared to the normal population
234. 15% of women with antiphospholipid antibodies suffer from recurrent miscarriage

A high head at term is associated with

235. Small angle of inclination of the pelvis
236. Afro-Caribbean race
237. Cephalopelvic disproportion

With regard to acute PID

238. It is generally caused by a sexually acquired pathogen
239. Penicillin and metronidazole are sufficient in treating the majority of infections
240. Bacterial vaginosis does not predispose to an increased risk
241. Up to 50% of women with gonococcal infection develop salpingitis

Progestogens

242. Medroxyprogesterone acetate is more androgenic than norethisterone
243. Levonorgestrel is more androgenic than norethisterone
244. Medroxyprogesterone increases oestradiol levels
245. 19-norsteroid derivatives have more deleterious effects on lipid profiles than medroxyprogesterone acetate
246. When used alone progestogens may halt bone-mineral loss in post-menopausal women

Regarding the Yuzpe method

247. It has a higher success rate in preventing unwanted pregnancy than IUCD used for post-coital contraception
248. It is contraindicated when unprotected intercourse has occurred with missed combined oral contraceptive pills

Small for gestational age neonates

249. Have excessive weight loss in the first 48 hours
250. Have increased liver glycogen storage
251. Have a body length less retarded than the body weight
252. In the UK make up over 50% of the low birth-weight babies
253. Have a decreased number of cells in each organ
254. Have an increased risk of hypothermia
255. Have an increased risk of hyperglycaemia
256. Have an increased risk of learning disorders in the long term

The following risk factors are positively correlated

257. Cervical carcinoma   Oral contraceptive pill
258. Ovarian carcinoma   Oral contraceptive pill
259. Endometrial carcinoma   Late menarche
260. Breast carcinoma   Levonorgestrel

In a newborn, cord blood measurements of Hb 13 g/dl, bilirubin 55 μmol/l and blood group B rhesus positive suggest

261. Rhesus incompatibility is the most likely diagnosis
262. The diagnosis could be ABO incompatibility
263. The direct bilirubin will be elevated
264. The residual albumin binding capacity will be low
265. The baby had an intrauterine transfusion within the previous 2 weeks

With regard to chemotherapy for trophoblastic disease

266. Methotrexate alone is the initial treatment
267. Following combined chemotherapy for resistant disease there is a risk of irreversible alopecia
268. Following combined chemotherapy for resistant disease there is a risk of acute myeloid leukaemia
269. Following combined chemotherapy for resistant disease there is a risk of colonic carcinoma

Cord prolapse is associated with

270. Increasing maternal age
271. Postmaturity
272. Circumvallate placenta
273. Prematurity
274. High parity
275. Keilland's forceps delivery
276. Multiple pregnancy

In radiotherapy for cervical carcinoma

277. Point A is 2 cm lateral from the cervical canal and 2 cm above the lateral vaginal fornices
278. Point B is 2 cm lateral from the midline and 5 cm above the lateral vaginal fornices

Diabetes and pregnancy

279. The incidence of diabetes mellitus in women of reproductive age is 0.3%
280. Currently the Caesarean delivery rate for diabetic women is 50%
281. Gestational diabetes is associated with increased incidence of fetal malformations
282. The hourly insulin dose for the 'sliding scale' is calculated by dividing the daily insulin dose in late pregnancy by 12

Anovulation is characteristically associated with

283. Turner's syndrome
284. Bulimia nervosa
285. Premenstrual tension
286. Sheehan's syndrome
287. Dysmenorrhoea

Neonatal jaundice occurring within 12 hours of birth may be caused by

288. Urinary tract infection
289. Bile duct atresia

In cervical cancer screening

290. The percentage of the population covered is an important contributing factor to the success of a screening program
291. Two thirds of women with invasive cervical cancer have never been screened
292. The incidence of cervical adenocarcinoma is falling due to the NHS screening programme
293. The reported frequency of false negative smears is up to 40%
294. The incidence of false negative smears is correlated with the size of the lesion

Treatment of bacterial vaginosis

295. Oral metronidazole 2 g as a single dose or 400 mg BD for 7 days could be used, 5 g of 2% clindamycin cream vaginally for 7 days is an alternative
296. Male partners should also be treated

Regarding urinary incontinence

297. Leaking urine is always an abnormal finding in healthy young women
298. Urinary incontinence is a condition of involuntary loss of urine
299. About 17% of women with urinary incontinence have a combination of genuine stress incontinence and detrusor instability
300. Clinical diagnosis is confirmed by urodynamics in 80–90% of cases

ANSWERS TO PAPER SIX

The numbers of the correct answers are given

Recognized causes of vaginal bleeding in an 8-year-old girl include
1, 2, 3, 8, 10   (Paediatric gynaecology)
Causes of vaginal bleeding may be secondary to cancer – sarcoma botryoides, foreign body, sexual abuse, rarely infection and precocious puberty, polyostotic fibrous dysplasia (Albright's syndrome), craniopharyngioma, and post-encephalitic syndrome. Wilson's disease is a recessively inherited disorder of copper metabolism.

Match
12, 13, 14
Overall, the 5 year survival for women with endometrial cancer is currently 65%.

Blood transfusion in pregnancy
15, 16
Blood transfusion in women with sickle cell disease improves blood and tissue oxygenation, and reduces the propensity for sickle cell crisis. Also, it temporarily suppresses production of new host red cells. Over-transfusion could lead to a hyperviscous state and increase the risk of sickle cell crisis. An increased risk of blood transfusion in women on aspirin has been suggested by the CLASP study, which demonstrated that the incidence of blood transfusion in women on low dose aspirin was higher than in the control group. This was thought to be a chance finding (rather than reliable evidence) as the incidence of post-partum haemorrhage was not increased.

References
CLASP Collaborative Group. CLASP: A randomised trial of low-dose aspirin for the prevention and treatment of pre-eclampsia among 9364 pregnant women. *Lancet*, 1994; **343**: 619–629.
De Swiet M. The use of low dose aspirin in pregnancy. RCOG PACE Review 96/03.
Howard RJ, Tuck SM. Sickle cell disease and pregnancy. *Current Obstetrics and Gynaecology*, 1995; **5**: 36–40.

Non-surgical management of urinary incontinence
20

Pelvic floor exercises are more successful in younger patients, because improved muscle tone is easier to achieve in this group. Faradism added to pelvic floor exercises does not confer a significant advantage when compared with pelvic floor exercises alone. Bladder drill is highly successful (up to 90% quoted), but the recurrence rate of urinary incontinence is high.

References

Barrington FW. The management of the urge syndrome. In: Studd J, ed. *Progress in Obstetrics and Gynaecology*, Volume 12. Edinburgh: Churchill Livingston, 1996; 259–276.

Cardozo L, Hill S. Urinary incontinence. RCOG PACE review 96/09.

Eckford SD, Keane D. Surgical treatment of urinary stress incontinence. *British Journal of Hospital Medicine*, 1992; **48**: 308–313.

Kelleher CJ, Cardozo LD. The conservative management of female urinary incontinence. *The Year Book of the RCOG* 1994; 123–135.

Richmond D. The incontinent woman: 1. *British Journal of Hospital Medicine*, 1993; **50**: 418–423.

Litigation
22

Preterm breech
23, 24, 25, 26   (Breech)

Vaginal delivery of the preterm breech is associated with an increased risk of cord prolapse due to a poor fit of the maternal pelvic soft tissue and fetal breech, and an increased risk of head entrapment due to a relatively large fetal head. Though prophylactic forceps delivery has been practised aiming to reduce trauma to the fetal head during its passage through the pelvis, there is no evidence of any benefit gained by this. At less than 28 weeks of pregnancy the mode of delivery does not make any difference to the degree of fetal trauma.

Reference

Penn ZJ. The preterm breech. *PACE review*. No 95/04.

The effect of pregnancy on cancer
29, 30, 33   (Cancer in pregnancy)

The prognosis of breast cancer when diagnosed in pregnancy is significantly worse because of the late diagnosis and higher chance of metastasis. Pregnancy has an adverse effect on the prognosis of melanoma.

Reference

Pregnancy after breast cancer. *RCOG Guideline* No 12, July 1997.

Regarding third generation combined oral contraceptive pills
35, 36
The risk of venous thrombo-embolism in desogestrel/gestodene pill users is half that in pregnancy. This is because third generation pills are associated with a lower risk of arterial disease, and as arterial disease produces 20-times higher mortality than venous thrombo-embolism, the use of third generation pills can be justified in this case. Changes can be considered if no second generation pill suits the woman, she does not want to take non-steroidal contraception, and understands and accepts the risk of thrombo-embolic complications associated with desogestrel/gestodene-containing pills.

Reference
Crook D. Do different brands of oral contraceptives differ in their effects on cardiovascular disease. *British Journal of Obstetrics and Gynaecology*, 1997; **104**: 516–520.

Perinatal mortality
39, 40, 41   (Perinatal mortality)
The perinatal mortality rate in the UK in the mid-1990s was 7–8 per 1000 total births. It is lowest for the social classes two and three, and is highest in social class five. The lowest PMR has been demonstrated in mothers 25–29 years old and is higher in teenagers and women of an advanced age. Other factors associated with perinatal mortality rate are birth weight, race, maternal health, smoking and maternal education. This is a multi-factorial parameter with a significant contribution from social and organizational factors. It has different definitions in different countries and improved neonatal care has made a significant contribution.

Reference
Whitfield CR. Vital statistics and derived information for obstetricians. In: CR Whitfield ed. *Dewhurst's Textbook of Obstetrics and Gynaecology for Postgraduates*, 5th edn. Blackwell Science, 1995; 494–510.

Hyperplasia
45, 47
Adenomatous is complex hyperplasia; simple is cystic (glandular) hyperplasia. The risk of developing endometrial cancer in a woman with a simple endometrial hyperplasia is 1% in 15 years.

References
Anderson MC, Robboy J. Aetiology and histopathology of endometrial hyperplasia and carcinoma. *Current Obstetrics and Gynaecology*, 1997; **7**: 2–7.
Oram DH, Jeyarajah AR. Diagnosis and management of endometrial hyperplasia. *Current Obstetrics and Gynaecology*, 1997; **7**: 8–15.

Post-partum haemorrhage
48, 49   (Post-partum haemorrhage)
Syntometrine is more effective than oxytocin when used alone.

Reference
Ekeroma A, Ansary A, Stirrat GM. Management of primary postpartum haemorrhage. *British Journal of Obstetrics and Gynaecology*, 1997; **104**: 275–277.

The risks associated with diabetes in pregnancy
51, 52, 55   (Diabetes and pregnancy)
The prevalence of pre-eclampsia is 14%, and preterm labour 17%.

References
Johnstone FD. Pregnancy management in women with insulin-dependent diabetes. *British Journal of Hospital Medicine*, 1997; **58**: 207–210.
Pearson JF. Pregnancy and complicated diabetes. *British Journal of Hospital Medicine*, 1993; **49**: 739–742.
Vaughan NJA. Diabetes in pregnancy. *Current Obstetrics and Gynaecology*, 1994; **4**: 155–159.

Regarding post-coital contraception
57, 58
The LNG-IUD is more expensive and more difficult to insert than a copper coil. It has not been evaluated as a post-coital contraceptive device.

The following are associated with endometrial cancer
59, 60, 61, 62   (Uterine tumours)
Unopposed oestrogen, obesity and nulliparity are also associated.

Reference
Semple D. Endometrial cancer. *British Journal of Hospital Medicine*, 1997; **57**(6): 260–262.

Caesarean delivery
64, 67   (Caesarean section)
Vaginal delivery after two previous Caesarean sections is possible and there is evidence to suggest that it is safe. It is possible to combine a Pfannenstiel incision with any type of uterine incision.

Vesico-vaginal fistula may be caused by
68, 69, 70
The commonest cause is iatrogenic.

Fetal effect of analgesia in labour
71, 73
Regional analgesia is associated with fetal heart rate decelerations due to reduced placental blood flow secondary to reduced peripheral resistance, whilst opioids pass through the placental barrier and have a direct effect on the fetal heart. Naloxone may become necessary if neonatal respiration is depressed due to high dose opioid administration in labour. It should not be used routinely because it may precipitate withdrawal in babies born to opiate addicts.

References

Enkin M, Keirse MJNC, Renfrew M, Neilson J. *A Guide to Effective Care in Pregnancy and Childbirth*, 2nd edn. Oxford: Oxford University Press, 1995; 247–261.

Morgan B. Maternal anaesthesia and analgesia in labour. In: James DK, Steer PJ, Weiner CP, Gonik B eds. *High Risk Pregnancy Management Options*. London: WB Saunders Company, 1994; 1101–1118.

Hydatidiform mole may present with

74, 75, 76   (Gestational trophoblastic disease)

Might present with hyperemesis, recurrent vaginal bleeding, hypertension, fitting and memory loss (Wernicke's encephalopathy – from thiamine deficiency)

Risk of thrombo-embolic disease and pregnancy

78, 81, 82, 83   (Coagulation and pregnancy)

The risk of thrombo-embolism in pregnancy is increased 6-fold. Other risk factors include maternal age over 35 years, obesity, grand multiparity, gross varicose veins, pre-eclampsia and operative delivery. The measurement of arterial blood gases for the diagnosis of pulmonary embolism has low sensitivity and specificity.

References

Report on Confidential Enquiries into Maternal Deaths in the United Kingdom, 1991–1993. London: HMSO, 1996.

Report of the RCOG Working Party on Prophylaxis against thromboembolism in Gynaecology and Obstetrics. March 1995.

Ray JG, Ginsberg JS. Thromboembolic disease during pregnancy: A practical guide for obstetricians. In: J Bonner ed. *Recent Advances in Obstetrics and Gynaecology*. 1995; 63–75.

Delayed puberty

85, 86, 91   (Menarche)

Associated with hyperprolactinaemia. Anorexia nervosa is not a common cause. Pulsatile GnRH can be used for treatment.

Endometriosis

94, 95, 96   (Endometriosis)

The commonest symptoms associated with mild endometriosis are congestive dysmenorrhoea, deep dyspareunia and pelvic pain. Viable endometrial cells found in peritoneal fluid at the time of menstruation may suggest that retrograde menstruation could be a cause. The exact aetiology remains a mystery. Endometriotic deposits often only contain progestin receptors found in lower concentrations than normal endometrium. Fallopian tubes should only be removed (to improve success rates prior to IVF) if there are bilateral hydrosalpinges, which are not often found with endometriosis.

Reference

Odukoya OA, Cooke ID. Endometriosis: a review. In: J Studd ed. *Progress in Obstetrics and Gynaecology*. **12**: 327–345.

Match the drugs to the correct side effects when used in late pregnancy

98, 101   (Epilepsy in pregnancy)

Hydralazine causes a tachycardia. Phenytoin does not cause congenital abnormality in late pregnancy.

Reference
British National Formulary. **35**; March 1998.

With regard to ovarian cancer

102   (Ovarian tumours: epithelial)

75% present with stage 3 to 4 disease.

Hyperprolactinaemia can be caused by

104, 105, 106, 108   (Hyperprolactinaemia)

Quinagolide is a treatment.

Maternal mortality

109, 110, 113

Maternal mortality over the age of 40 years was 20.6 per 100 000 maternity (1991–93). Avoidable factors were present in 44.6% of cases (1985–93). Thromboembolism is the biggest single cause.

Reference
Report on Confidential Enquiries into Maternal Deaths in the United Kingdom, 1991–1993. London: HMSO, 1996.

Treatment of CIN

115, 116, 121, 123   (Premalignant disease of the cervix)

Among excisional biopsy techniques, the cone biopsy is the most traumatic but has the highest success rate – over 90%. The quality of material for histological diagnosis obtained by laser excision is no better than that obtained by loop diathermy or knife conization. CGIN is characterized by skip lesions, therefore clear margins of excision cannot guarantee complete excision. Local ablative techniques do not provide material for histological diagnosis, therefore where severe dyskaryosis is present excisional biopsies are recommended. Amongst ablative treatment methods the CO_2 laser causes tissue destruction to a depth of 2–3 mm and cold coagulation to a depth of 3–4 mm. Cryocautery is the treatment of choice for small superficial lesions.

References
Houghton SJ, Luesley DM. LLETZ – diathermy loop excision. *Current Obstetrics and Gynaecology*, 1995; **5**: 107–109.
Shafi MI, Jordan JA. The treatment of CIN. *Current Obstetrics and Gynaecology*, 1991; **1**: 137–142.

Detrusor instability

Pelvic floor exercises and the bladder drill should be performed at the same time. This may lead to an improvement in symptoms making surgery unnecessary.

References

Cardozo L, Hill S. Urinary incontinence. RCOG PACE review 96/09.

Richmond D. The incontinent woman: 2. *British Journal of Hospital Medicine*, 1993; **50**: 490–492

Vulval carcinoma is associated with
125, 126, 127, 128   (Vulva)

References

Maclean AB. Precursors of vulval cancers. *Current Obstetrics and Gynaecology*, 1993; **3**: 149–156.

Evans S. Vulval skin disease and the gynaecologist. *British Journal of Hospital Medicine*, 1997; **57**: 579–581.

Sarhanis P, Blackett AD, Sharp F. Intraepithelial neoplasia of the anogenital area: a multicentric condition. *Current Obstetrics and Gynaecology*, 1996; **6**: 92–97.

Interactions of the combined oral contraceptive pill and other drugs
129, 130, 131

Twin pregnancy
132, 134, 135, 137, 138   (Multiple pregnancy)

The perinatal mortality of the second twin is higher. It is generally caused by fertilization of two ova by two sperms following one act of coitus (dizygotic) or division of the fertilized ovum (monozygotic). Superfecundation means fertilization of two ova with two sperms following two separate acts of coitus in the same cycle (rare). Monozygous twins may be dichorionic.

Reference

Neilson JP. Multiple pregnancy. In: Whitfield CR, ed. *Dewhurst's Textbook of Obstetrics and Gynaecology for Postgraduates*, 5th edn. Oxford: Blackwell Science, 1995; 439–453.

Management of endometrial cancer
145, 147

Transvaginal scanning is not of any proven value in the diagnosis of endometrial cancer in premenopausal women. Pipelle biopsy of endometrium offers the advantage of avoiding general (or regional) anaesthesia, the diagnosis is not necessarily achieved more rapidly. Endometrial cancer is a contraindication for endometrial resection at any stage. The current management of stage 1 endometrial cancer is controversial and some would argue that a radical hysterectomy is the treatment of choice, particularly for high grade tumours or deep myometrial invasion. The response to progestogen therapy is poorer the higher the grade of the tumour. Progestogen therapy is used in stage 4 endometrial cancer for palliation. Tamoxifen increases the number of progesterone receptors thus increasing the effectiveness of progesterone therapy. Extrapelvic disease is better treated with radiotherapy.

References

Buxton E.J. Surgical management of endometrial cancer. *Current Obstetrics and Gynaecology*, 1997; **7**: 16–21.

Horowitz IR, Shingleton HM. The role of chemotherapy and radiotherapy in the treatment of endometrial carcinoma. *Current Obstetrics and Gynaecology*, 1997; **7**: 22–29.

Lawton F. The management of endometrial cancer. *British Journal of Obstetrics and Gynaecology*, 1997; **104**: 127–134.

Woolas R, Oram D. Current developments in the management of endometrial cancer. In: *The Year Book of the RCOG 1994*; 181–193.

Uterine sarcomas
149

Reference

Olah KS, Kingston RE. Uterine sarcomas. *Progress in Obstetrics and Gynaecology*, **11**: 427–445.

Recognized associations of persistent ductus arteriosus in the neonate include
150, 152

It is not a feature of Marfan's syndrome (aortic regurgitation is common). After birth the blood will flow from the aorta towards the lungs if the ductus remains patent (due to high systemic resistance compared to low resistance of the pulmonary bed) leading to pulmonary hyperaemia. Prenatal administration of indomethacin is associated with premature closure of the ductus.

Reference

Whitfield CR. Heart disease in pregnancy. In: Whitfield CR, ed. *Dewhurst's Textbook of Obstetrics and Gynaecology for Postgraduates*, 5th edn. Oxford: Blackwell Science, 1995; 216–217.

Radiotherapy in the management of gynaecological cancer
155, 157   (Radiotherapy)

Although the success rates of surgery and radiotherapy are similar, the complication rate of radiotherapy is higher. Currently chemotherapy is preferred to radiotherapy for treatment of ovarian cancer as it has a lower complication rate. Exenterative surgery is the preferred mode of treatment of central pelvic recurrences. Brachytherapy is a type of radiotherapy with an intracavity radiation source.

References

Horowitz IR, Shingleton HM. The role of chemotherapy and radiotherapy in the treatment of endometrial carcinoma. *Current Obstetrics and Gynaecology*, 1997; **7**: 22–29.

Sproston ARM. Non-surgical treatment of cervical carcinoma. *British Journal of Hospital Medicine*, 1994; **52**: 30–34.

Viral infections of the genital tract

161, 162, 165 (Sexually transmitted disease)

Genital warts could be treated in pregnancy with electrocautery, laser or trichloroacetic acid. Podophyllin is contraindicated in pregnancy. In pregnancy, 50% of genital herpetic infections are caused by HSV1 and 50% by HSV2.

References

Crook T, Farthing A. Human papillomavirus and cervical cancer. *British Journal of Hospital Medicine*, 1993; **49**: 131–132.

Maclean AB, Macnab FCM. The role of viruses in gynaecological oncology. In: Studd J, ed. *Progress in Obstetrics and Gynaecology*, Volume 12. 1996; 403–417.

Stabile I, Chard T, Grudzinskas G. *Clinical Obstetrics and Gynaecology*. New York: Springer-Verlag 1996; 184.

Lymphogranuloma venereum

167, 168, 169

Tetracycline is the antibiotic of choice.

Predisposing factors for an ectopic pregnancy include

172, 173, 177 (Ectopic pregnancy)

The OCP is not associated with an increased risk. The risk increases as a result of exposure to diethylstilboestrol *in utero*. Artificial insemination is not associated with a higher risk, but IVF, GIFT etc., are. Chlamydia is associated with it, not candida.

The following match

In the UK candidiasis and bacterial vaginosis and candida infection are commoner than trichomonal infection. Greenish vaginal discharge is characteristic of trichomonal infection, whilst bacterial vaginosis commonly has a greyish discharge. Chlamydia is rarely associated with a colourless, odourless discharge; candidiasis is associated with the thick white discharge described.

References

Emens JM. Intractable vaginal discharge. *Current Obstetrics and Gynaecology*, 1993; **3**: 41–47.

Lamont RF. Bacterial vaginosis. *The Year Book of the RCOG 1994*. 149–158.

Thomas EJ, Rock J. *Benign Gynaecological Disease*. Oxford: Health Press. 1997, 52–58.

Vaginal adenosis

182

GSI
183   (Urinary incontinence: urodynamics)
Topical oestrogen application could be an effective therapy for GSI in post-menopausal women.

References
Bidmean J, Cardozo L. Detrusor instability. RCOG PACE review 98/03.
Cardozo L, Hill S. Urinary incontinence. RCOG PACE review 96/09.

Perinatal medicine
186, 187   (Perinatal mortality)
The terms used for classifying birth weight are: low birth weight < 2500 g; very low birth weight < 1500 g; extremely low birth weight < 1000 g.

Mifepristone
189, 190, 193   (Therapeutic abortion)
Mifepristone is an antiprogestogen. It has antiglucocorticoid action and is contra-indicated in women with prolonged systemic steroid administration or chronic adrenal failure. Other contraindications include smoking in those over 35 years of age, haemorrhagic disorders, and when ectopic pregnancy is not ruled out.

References
British National Formulary. **36**; March 1998.
Henshaw RC, Templeton AA. Methods used in first trimester abortion. *Current Obstetrics and Gynaecology*, 1993; **3**: 11–16.

Medical termination of pregnancy is associated with
195   (Therapeutic abortion)
Although with medical management the incidence of complete abortion is 95%, the incidence of ongoing pregnancy is less than 1%. Therefore, adequate follow-up is very important to rule out retained products of pregnancy or a viable pregnancy.

Reference
Henshaw RC, Templeton AA. Methods used in first trimester abortion. *Current Obstetrics and Gynaecology*, 1993; **3**: 11–16.

Pre-eclampsia
197, 200   (Pre-eclampsia, eclampsia and phaeochromocytoma)
It is diagnosed after 20 weeks by definition. Diazepam is not contraindicated. The criteria for diagnosis are hypertension and proteinuria (not albuminuria).

Reference
Redman C. Hypertension in pregnancy. In: De Swiet M, ed. *Medical Disorders in Obstetrics Practice*, 2nd edn. Oxford: Blackwell Science, 1990; 249–305.

Klinefelter's syndrome is associated with
201
Other features include tall height, small testes, gynaecomastia, educational difficulties without any major shift in IQ score etc. The incidence is 1 in 600 at birth. Kartagener's syndrome is associated with dextrocardia and infertility.

Reference
Neilson JP. Antenatal diagnosis of fetal abnormality. In: Whitfield CR, ed. *Dewhurst's Textbook of Obstetrics and Gynaecology for Postgraduates*, 5th edn, Oxford: Blackwell Science, 1995; 121–139.

Predisposing factors for ARDS are
203
It is associated with general anaesthesia.

Reference
Craft TM, Upton PM, eds. *Key topics in Anaesthesia*. Oxford: BIOS Scientific Publishers, 1993; 19–21.

The management of a woman in pregnancy with a history of herpes infection (but with no visible lesions at present) includes
206, 207   (Infection in pregnancy)
Weekly cultures are not cost effective. A Caesarean section is indicated only in the presence of active lesion. The incidence of neonatal herpes is 2:100 000 live births in the UK (1:3000 to 1:20 000 live births in USA). Up to 60% of babies with neonatal herpes are born to mothers with no symptoms or signs of the disease at delivery. The infection is neither notifiable nor requires isolation. The risk of neonatal herpes is 50% with primary attack in the mother at delivery and 5% with recurrent attack at delivery. The mortality is 60% in the affected neonates. Vidarabine and acyclovir improve survival in neonatal herpes, but the survivors with herpes encephalitis have severe neurological impairment.

Reference
Pregnancy and the neonate. In: Adler MW, Weller I, Goldmeier D, eds. *ABC of Sexually Transmitted Diseases*, 2nd edn. London: BMJ Publishing Group, 1990; 57–60.

Spermicides
210, 211, 212   (Contraception and sterilization)

Reference
Smith C. Barrier methods. Contraception. In: *Contraception*. Edition 95, 33–36. Reed Healthcare Communications.

Regarding HIV infection the following are true
215, 217, 218, 219 (Infection in pregnancy)
26% of pregnant women with HIV get infected through IV drug abuse (themselves or their partners), 58% of mothers are infected heterosexually from abroad; only 6% have no risk factors. Pregnancy appears to have no deleterious effects upon HIV disease. Transmission rates vary but are reported to be 25–30% in Europe. Postnatal transmission rates of up to 60% have been described in Africa. When mothers acquire the infection postnatally the risks of transmission are 29%. Avoiding breastfeeding can reduce the rates by half, and anti-retroviral therapy can further reduce it by two thirds. Caesarean section may also reduce it. Overall, using these measures rates can be reduced to 5–8%. Kaposi's sarcoma is a rare presentation. Anal intercourse is associated with a twofold increased risk of acquiring HIV from an infected man, vaginal intercourse is a lower risk activity. Using barrier methods and/or spermicides (Nonoxynol) can reduce transmission during sexual intercourse. Sperm donors are screened twice before their semen is released for use; this reduces but does not eliminate the risk.

References
Mercey, D. Antenatal HIV testing. *BMJ*, 1998; **316**: 241-242.
Norman S, Johnson M, Studd J. HIV infection in women. In: Studd J, ed. *Progress in Obstetrics and Gynaecology*, Volume 10. Edinburgh: Churchill Livingstone, 1993; 231–246.

Preterm labour
221, 222, 224 (Premature labour)
There is no evidence that the use of ritodrine improves perinatal outcome. Its use is recommended to delay delivery for 48 hours for the steroids to act. Epidural analgesia is not contraindicated.

The expulsion rate of IUCD is higher
226 (Contraception and sterilization)

Regarding postoperative complications
229 (Perioperative complications)
Pelvic cysts can also occur as lymph collections.

Recurrent miscarriage
232, 233 (Abortion spontaneous/recurrent)
Paternal chromosomal abnormalities are only found in 5% of couples. Polycystic ovaries are found in 56% compared with a background incidence of 22% (the background incidence of PCOS is 2%). 15% of women suffering from recurrent miscarriage have persistently elevated titres of antiphospholipid antibodies.

Reference
Rai R, Regan L. The management of recurrent miscarriage. PACE Review No 96/08.

A high head at term is associated with
236, 237   (Cephalopelvic disproportion)
The other associations of the high head at term are low-lying placenta, pelvic mass, high angle of inclination.

With regard to acute PID
238   (Pelvic inflammatory disease)
Penicillin and metronidazole are inadequate treatments, they will not eradicate chlamydia which is responsible for the majority of cases of PID in the UK (erythromycin or a tetracycline is indicated). Bacterial vaginosis does predispose to an increased risk. 10–20% of women with gonococcal infection develop salpingitis.

Progestogens
244, 245, 246
Medroxyprogesterone acetate and dydrogesterone are less androgenic than norethisterone and levonorgestrel. Medroxyprogesterone acetate reduces levels of SHBG which increases free oestradiol.

Reference
Pickersgill A. GnRH analogues and add-back therapy. Is there a perfect combination? *British Journal of Obstetrics and Gynaecology*, 1998; **105**: 475-485.

Regarding the Yuzpe method
The reverse is true for the IUCD. It should be used when a pill has been missed at the start of a cycle.

Reference
Glasier A. Emergency contraception and RU486. In: *Contraception*. Edition 95, 44–45. Reed Healthcare Communications.

Small for gestational age neonates
251, 254, 256
They have excessive heat loss in the first 48 hours. The glycogen content of the liver is less, predisposing them to hypoglycaemia. The commonest cause of low birth-weight babies in the UK is prematurity. The majority of the small for gestational age neonates have a normal number of cells in each organ (except in cases of symmetric growth restriction affecting the fetus in the phase of cellular hyperplasia).

References
Common disorders of the newborn infant. In: Johnson PGB, ed. Vulliamy's *The Newborn Child*, 7th edn. Edinburgh: Churchill Livingstone, 1994; 69–82.
Pearce JM, Robinson G. Fetal growth and growth retardation. In: Chamberlain G, ed. *Turnbull's Obstetrics*, 2nd edn. Edinburgh: Churchill Livingstone, 1995; 299–312.

The following risk factors are positively correlated
257
The oral contraceptive pill protects against ovarian carcinoma. Like ovarian carcinoma, endometrial carcinoma is associated with an early menarche and late menopause. There is no convincing evidence to link breast carcinoma to levonorgestrel.

In a newborn cord blood measurements of Hb 13 gm/dl, bilirubin 55 μmol/l and blood group B rhesus positive suggest
261, 262, 264

Reference
Jaundice in the newborn infant. In: Chamberlain GVP, ed. *Obstetrics by Ten Teachers*, 16th edn. London: Edward Arnold, 1995; 325–327.

With regard to chemotherapy for trophoblastic disease
268, 269   (Gestational trophoblastic disease)
Methotrexate is used in combination with folinic acid. The alopecia is reversible. There is also an increased risk of breast carcinoma following combined chemotherapy for resistant disease.

Reference
Newlands E.S. Trophoblastic disease. RCOG PACE review 96/10.

Cord prolapse is associated with
273, 274, 275, 276
Other causes are breech presentation (6%, 40–50% of all cord prolapse), rupture of the membranes with a high head, transverse lie, brow and face presentation, occipito-posterior position, cephalopelvic disproportion, manual rotation of head, vellamentous insertion of cord etc. Incidence is 1/200–300 deliveries.

Reference
Ritchie JWK. Malpositions of the occiput and malpresentations. In: Whitfield CR, ed. *Dewhurst's Textbook of Obstetrics and Gynaecology for Postgraduates*, 5th edn. Oxford: Blackwell Science, 1995; 346–367.

In radiotherapy for cervical carcinoma
278   (Radiotherapy)
Point B is 5 cm lateral from the midline and 2 cm above the lateral vaginal fornices.

Reference
Sproston ARM. Non-surgical treatment of cervical carcinoma. *British Journal of Hospital Medicine*, 1994; **52**: 30–34

Diabetes and pregnancy
279   (Diabetes and pregnancy)
The Caesarean section rate in women with diabetes mellitus is 30%. Gestational diabetes gradually develops during pregnancy and does not impose any threat to the fetal formation process. The hourly dose of insulin should be calculated by dividing pre-labour daily dose of insulin by 24.

References
Johnstone FD. Pregnancy management in women with insulin-dependent diabetes. *British Journal of Hospital Medicine*, 1997; **58**: 207–210.
Pearson JF. Pregnancy and complicated diabetes. *British Journal of Hospital Medicine*, 1993; **49**: 739–742.
Vaughan NJA. Diabetes in pregnancy. *Current Obstetrics and Gynaecology*, 1994; **4**: 155–159.

Anovulation is characteristically associated with
283, 286   (Infertility – I)
Anovulation is associated with anorexia nervosa. Premenstrual tension occurs in ovulatory cycles. It is not a cause of dysmenorrhoea.

Neonatal jaundice occurring within 12 hours of birth may be caused by
288
Bile duct atresia takes longer to develop into jaundice.

Reference
Jaundice in the newborn infant. In: Chamberlain GVP, ed. *Obstetrics by Ten Teachers*, 16th edn. London: Edward Arnold, 1995; 325–327.

In cervical cancer screening
290, 291, 294   (Premalignant disease of the cervix)
The cervical screening programme was started in 1988. Although there have been significant falls in the incidence of squamous cell carcinoma of the cervix (7% a year) the incidence of adenocarcinoma has not fallen. The frequency of false negative smears is reported to be 2–20%.

Reference
Patnick J. Has screening for cervical cancer been successful? *British Journal of Obstetrics and Gynaecology*, 1997; **104**: 876–878

Treatment of bacterial vaginosis
295
No benefit from treatment of the male partner has been demonstrated.

References

Lamont RF. Bacterial vaginosis. *The Year Book of the RCOG 1994*; 149–158.

MacDermott RIJ. Bacterial Vaginosis. *British Journal of Obstetrics and Gynaecologists* 1995; **102**: 92–94.

Regarding urinary incontinence

299   (Urinary incontinence: urodynamics)

Urinary incontinence should be objectively demonstrable, and cause social and hygiene problems to qualify as such. Up to 50% of healthy women leak urine occasionally. This does not cause hygienic or social problems and therefore does not need investigating or treating. The majority of studies suggest that urodynamics confirms the clinical diagnosis in 55–75% of cases.

References

Bidmean J, Cardozo L. Detrusor instability. RCOG PACE review 98/03.

Cardozo L, Hill S. Urinary incontinence. RCOG PACE review 96/09.

Jarvis GJ. Female urinary incontinence - which patients? - which tests?. *The Year Book of the RCOG 1994*; 111–120.

Richmond D. The incontinent woman: 1. *British Journal of Hospital Medicine*, 1993; **50**: 418–423.

Richmond D. The incontinent woman: 2. *British Journal of Hospital Medicine*, 1993; **50**: 490–492.

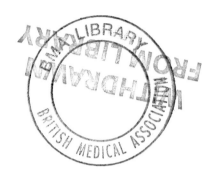